YOGA
for Vital Beauty

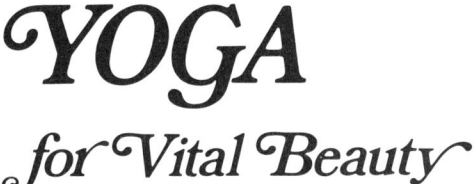

YOGA
for Vital Beauty

by Swami : Sarasvati

and Sadhu the Cat

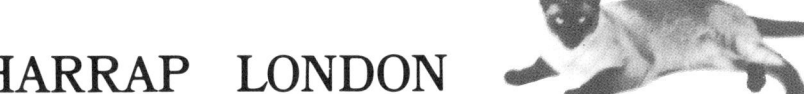

HARRAP   LONDON

Published in Australia 1970
by Horwitz Publications

© *Swami Sarasvati* 1970

First published in Great Britain 1972
by George G. Harrap & Co. Ltd
182-184 High Holborn, London WC1V 7AX

Reprinted 1975 ; 1978

ISBN 0 245 50995 X

Printed in Great Britain by
Redwood Burn Limited
Trowbridge & Esher

Made in Great Britain

Introduction

The asanas (exercises) in this book are the ones
I have found most popular with my television audience.
They are divided into sections according to the part
of the body each one affects and are *not* set out in
order of difficulty. It doesn't matter which one you try
first or whether or not you complete the entire movement.
Simply do as much as you can, even if it's only the
first stage.

Breathing, gentle exercise and a little relaxation each day
will not only reveal your inner beauty but will also give
you a firm body and a healthy mental outlook. You will
develop a more positive approach to living and become
more energetic, active and younger looking. (Would you
believe I am forty? I don't look more than sixteen do I!)

Once you begin practising yoga you will never stop,
because yoga is fun and enjoyable. Yoga is never
strenuous, its movements are gentle, especially designed
to rid your body of muscular and mental tension.

Remember, relaxation is beauty, tension is ugliness.

Swami Sarasvati

Contents

Breathing and Stretching

Breathing

Pranayama—Breath control

Breath is life and no one has realised this more than the Yogis of India to whom deep, controlled, rhythmic breathing is the first of all *Asanas* (exercises)

Correct breathing releases tension, improves digestion, cures constipation, and keeps you looking, and feeling, younger.

Relaxation Breath

Even in breathing we begin with relaxation.

Sitting cross-legged, or in the lotus position (as in the photograph), join your index finger and thumb and lower your chin till it rests in the notch between your collarbones, on top of the breastbone. Slowly breathe in and out.

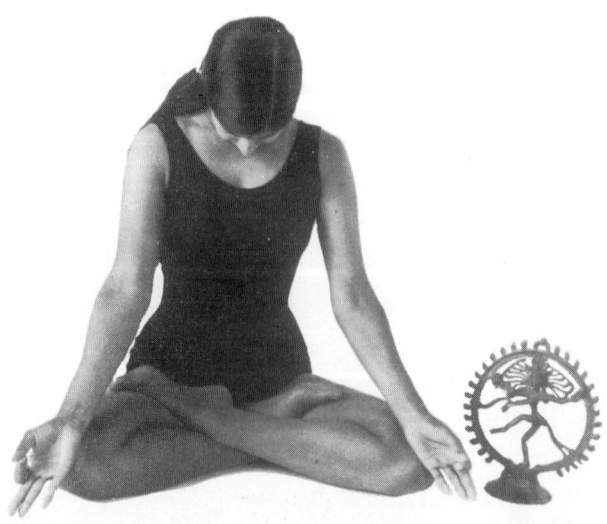

Three Stages of the Complete Yoga Breath

The lungs are long organs running from the collarbone to the diaphragm and yoga insists we breathe fully, filling and emptying the lungs completely—the lower part *(diaphragm or tummy breathing)*; the middle part *(chest breathing)*; and finally the upper part under the collarbone *(shoulder breathing)*.

Concentrate on practising the three stages until you are able to do them in one rhythmic, flowing movement.

Breathing with the Diaphragm (usually one of the most neglected breathing exercises)

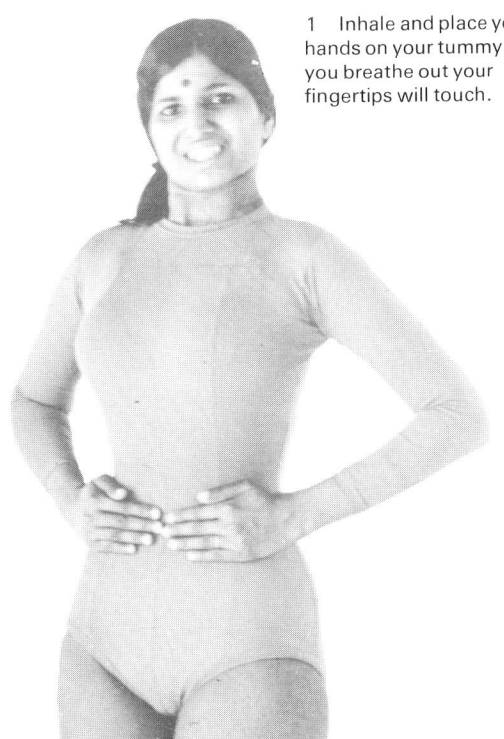

1   Inhale and place your hands on your tummy. As you breathe out your fingertips will touch.

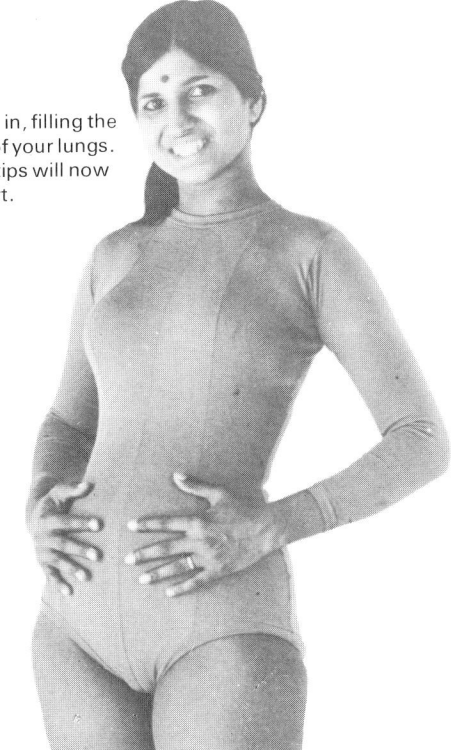

2   Breathe in, filling the lower part of your lungs. Your fingertips will now spread apart.

Chest Breathing

Chest breathing is the way we usually breathe, but we will now try breathing more slowly and deeply.

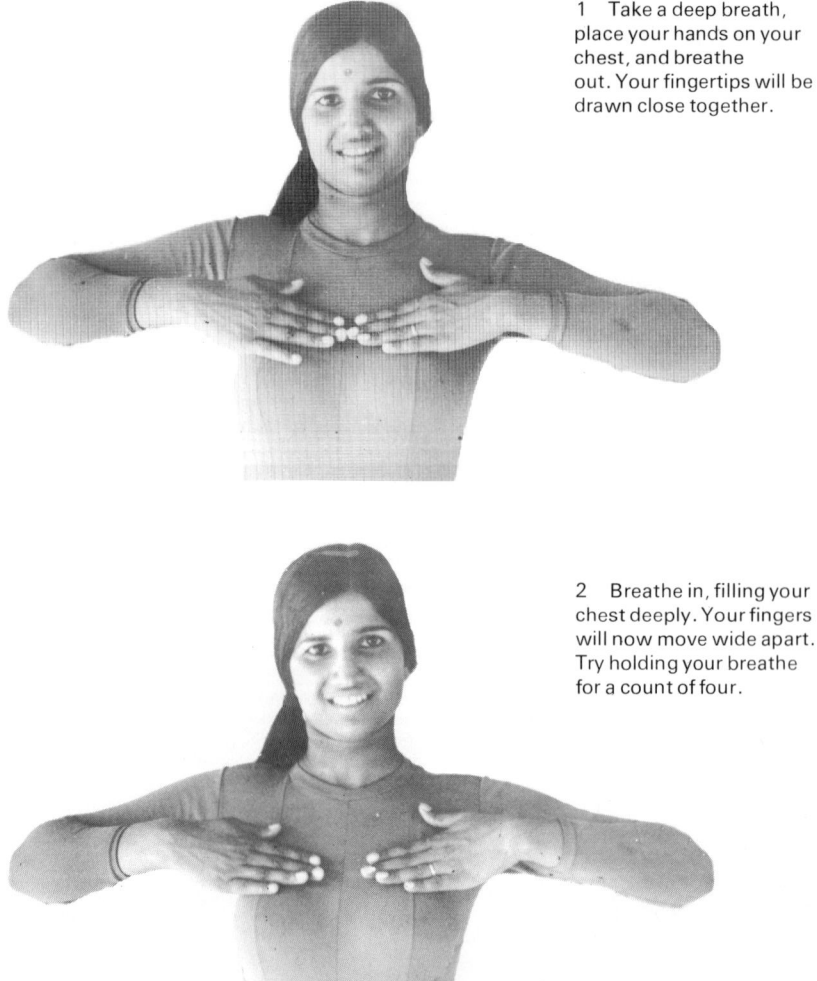

1   Take a deep breath, place your hands on your chest, and breathe out. Your fingertips will be drawn close together.

2   Breathe in, filling your chest deeply. Your fingers will now move wide apart. Try holding your breathe for a count of four.

Upper, or Shoulder, Breathing

As you inhale, fill your mind and body with positive thoughts of energy and strength; and as you breathe out, banish negative thoughts of sickness and worry.

1   Elbows bent, fingertips touching in front of your chest.

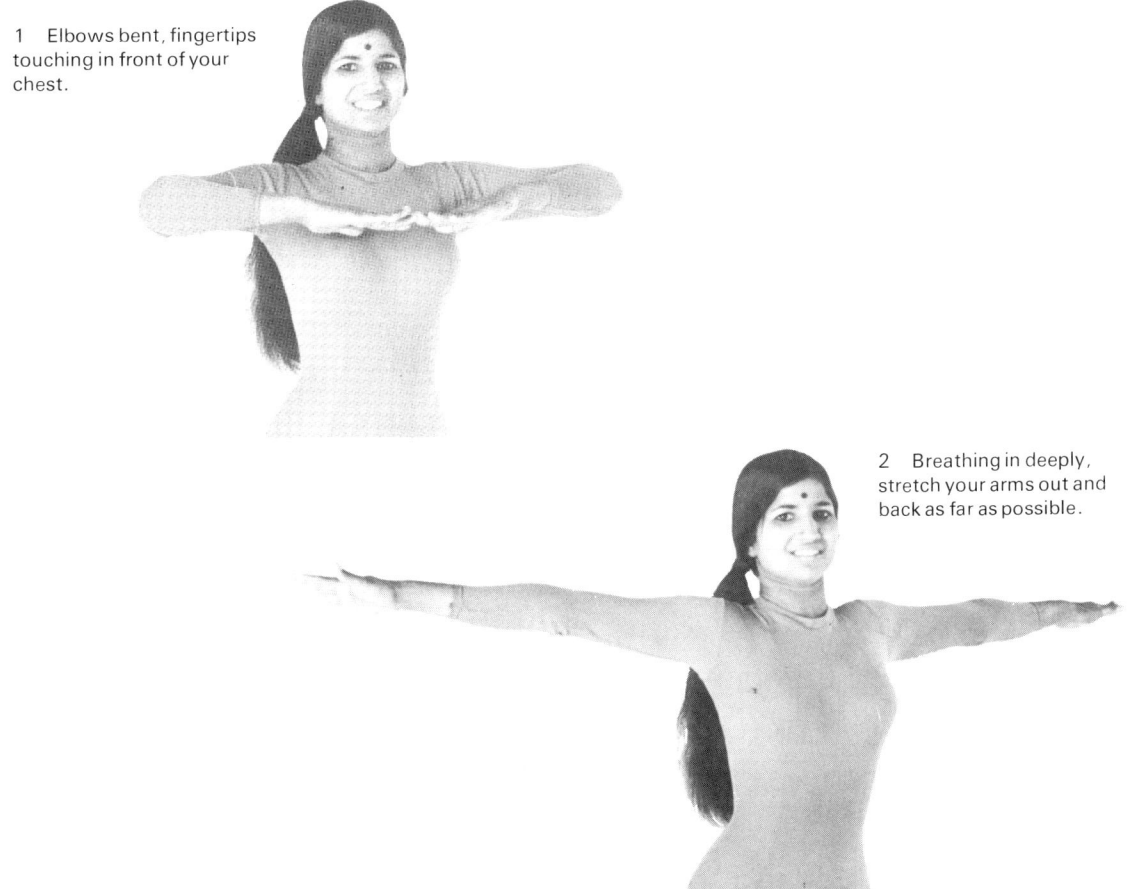

2   Breathing in deeply, stretch your arms out and back as far as possible.

Alternate Nostril Breathing

Let us take a deep breath and pray to God that we may rise above failure, frustration and discouragement, and have another try at making the most of our lives.

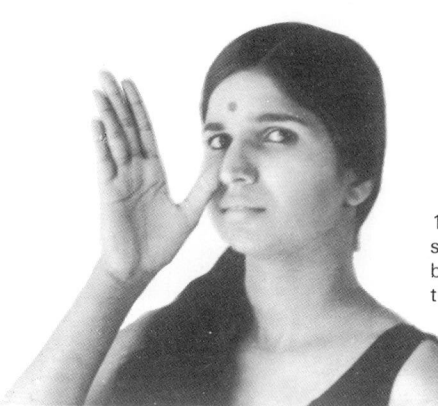

1   Sit with your back straight and shoulders back. Place your right thumb on your right nostril.

2   Two fingers between your eyebrows, and your third finger on your left nostril; open your left nostril and *inhale*. Close both nostrils and *hold your breath* for the count of four. Now open your right nostril and *exhale*. *Inhale* through your right nostril, *hold your breath* for the count of four and then *exhale* through your left nostril. This completes one cycle of alternate nostril breathing.

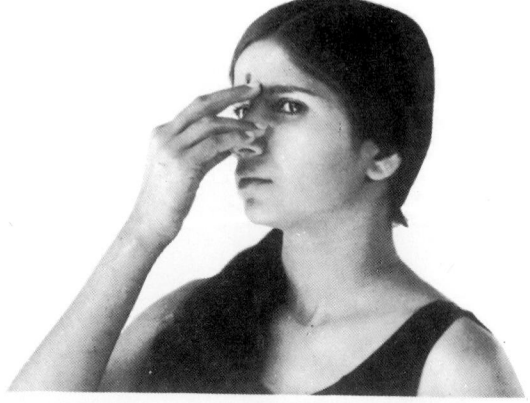

Stretching

Four Way Stretch

Stretch often. In the morning it awakens the body, during the day it releases tension, and stretching at night helps you to sleep.

1   Stand with your feet slightly apart and breathing in, stretch your hands above your head, stretching your entire body at the same time.

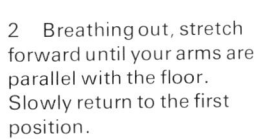

2   Breathing out, stretch forward until your arms are parallel with the floor. Slowly return to the first position.

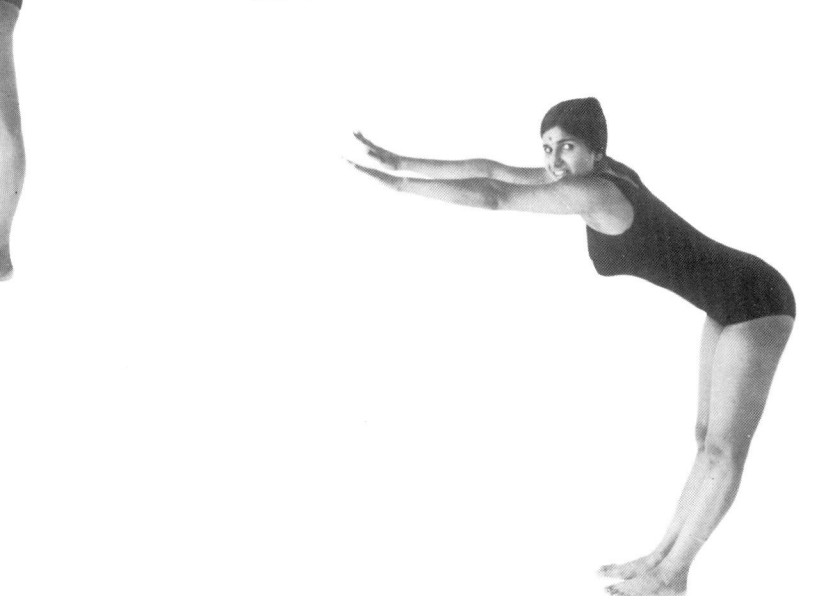

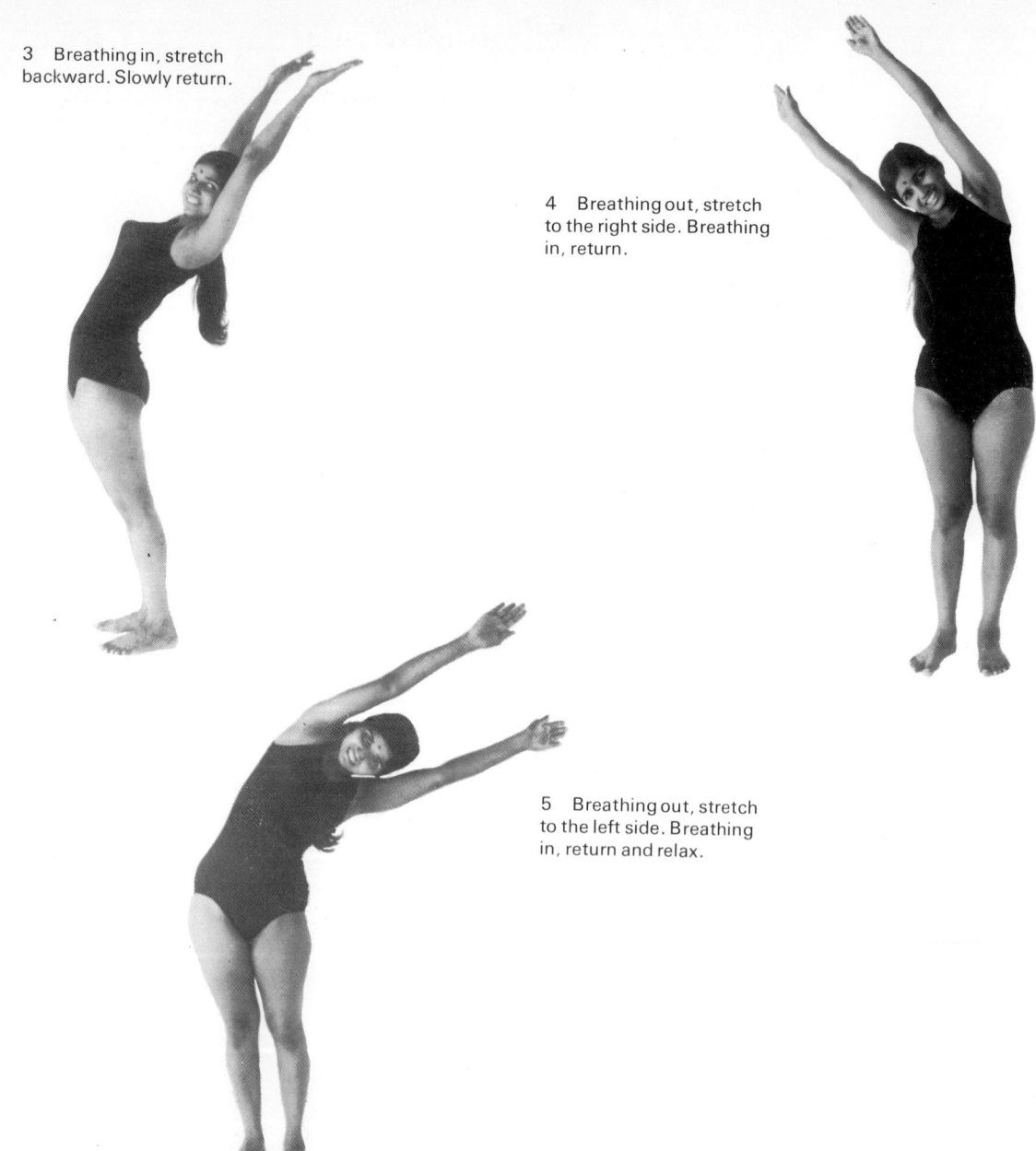

3 Breathing in, stretch backward. Slowly return.

4 Breathing out, stretch to the right side. Breathing in, return.

5 Breathing out, stretch to the left side. Breathing in, return and relax.

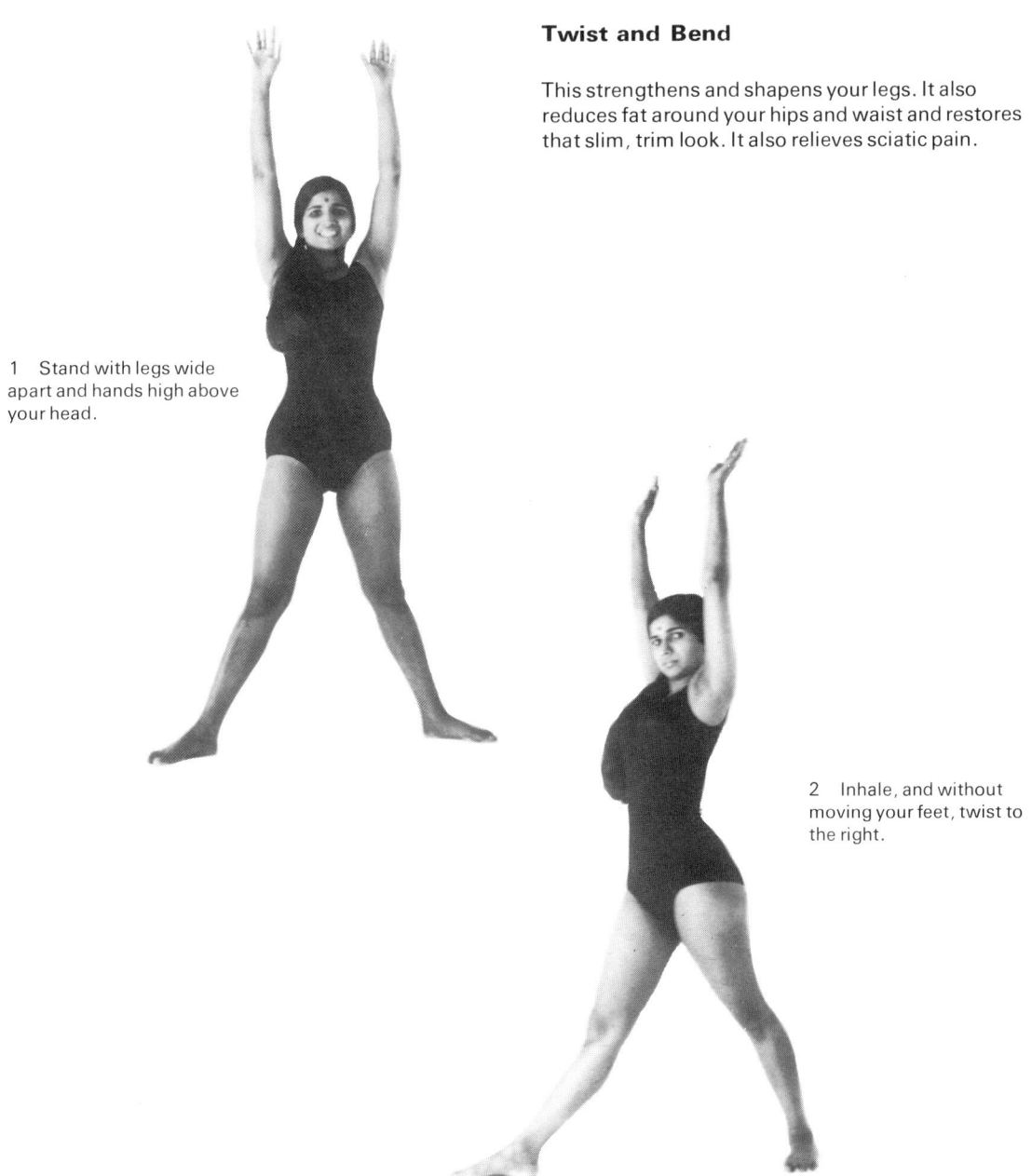

Twist and Bend

This strengthens and shapens your legs. It also reduces fat around your hips and waist and restores that slim, trim look. It also relieves sciatic pain.

1   Stand with legs wide apart and hands high above your head.

2   Inhale, and without moving your feet, twist to the right.

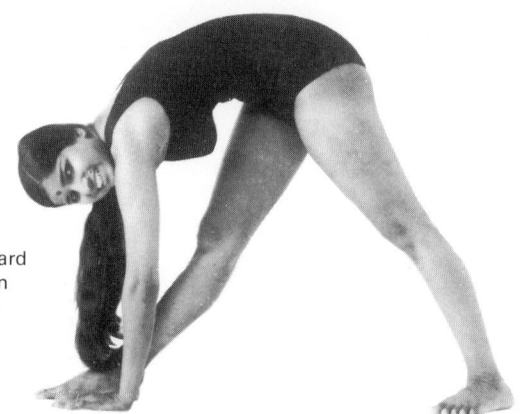

3　Exhaling, lean forward and place your palms on either side of your right foot.

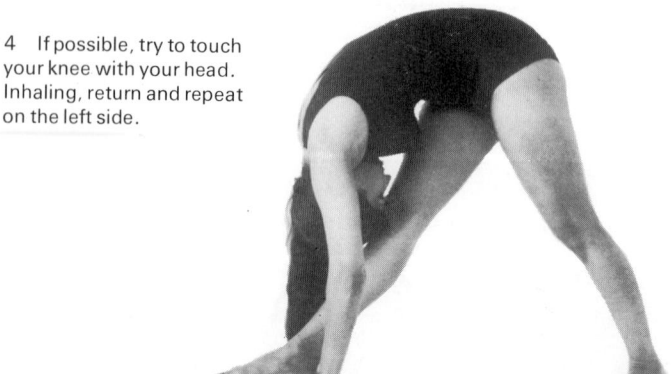

4　If possible, try to touch your knee with your head. Inhaling, return and repeat on the left side.

Walking on all Fours

An excellent way to make your spine supple and elastic.
Slims and reshapes your legs, thighs and hips.
Removes tension from the back of your legs making
them youthful and firm. It also relieves heel pains.

1   Place your palms on
the floor, keeping your
knees straight if possible.

2   Take a small step
forward with your right
hand and then with your
left hand.

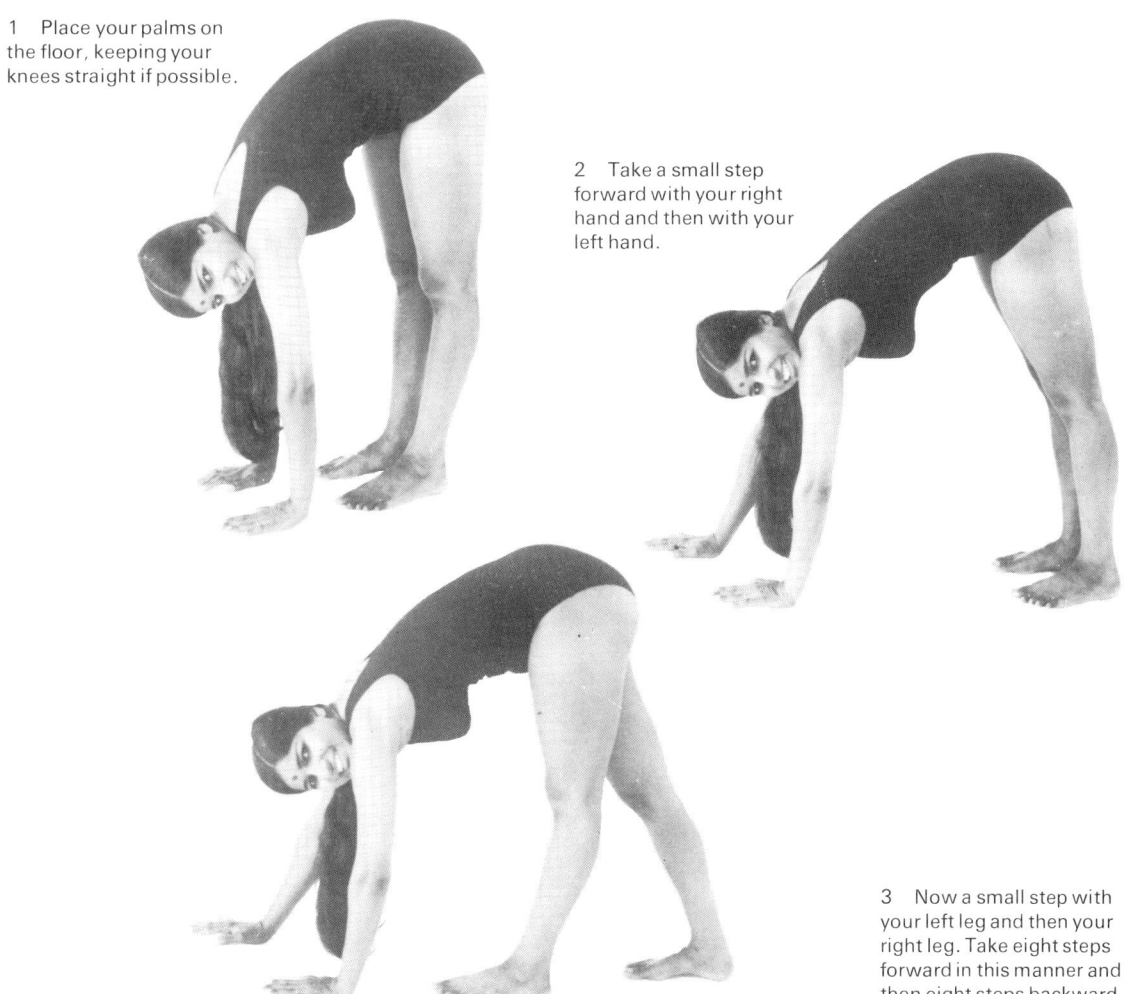

3   Now a small step with
your left leg and then your
right leg. Take eight steps
forward in this manner and
then eight steps backward.

Back Bend

Forward and backward bending delays aging of the lower back region.

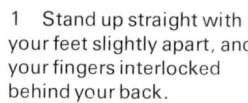
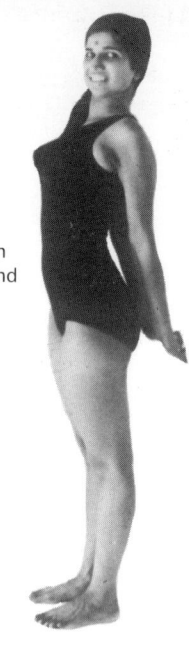

1   Stand up straight with your feet slightly apart, and your fingers interlocked behind your back.

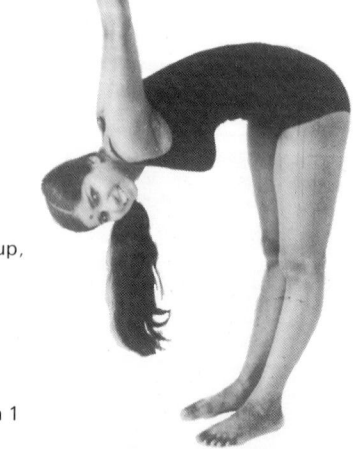

2   **Inhaling,** gently push your hips forward.

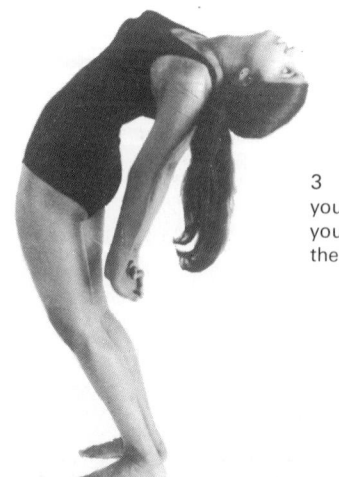

3   Still breathing in, drop your head back and push your hands down towards the floor.

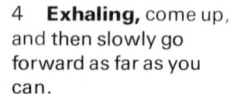

4   **Exhaling,** come up, and then slowly go forward as far as you can.

5   Return to position 1 and relax.

1 Stand straight, feet slightly apart, hands on your chest in prayer position.

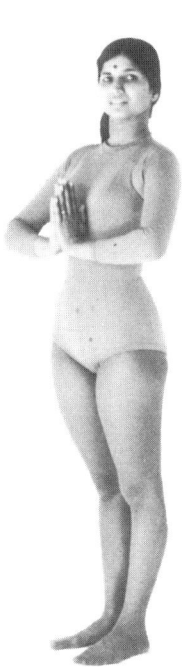

Surya Namaskar (Salute to the Sun)

The 12 steps of this ancient movement will not only tone all the muscles of your body, keep your joints supple and restore your glands to youthful vitality, but will also give you a positive attitude towards your day's work.

2 **Inhaling,** raise your hands above your head. As you become more supple you will be able to stretch your hands and body backwards at the same time.

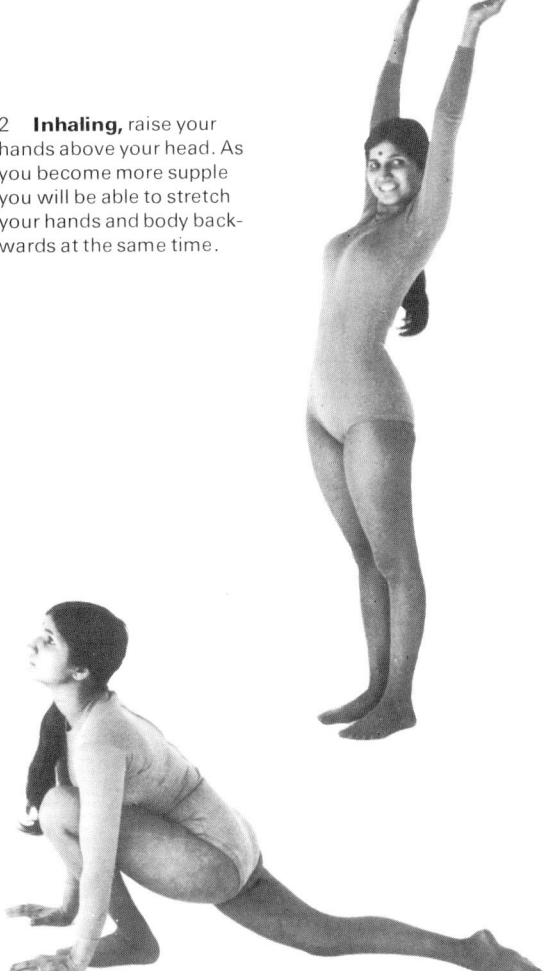

3 **Exhaling,** bend forward until your hands touch the ground. Keep your knees straight.

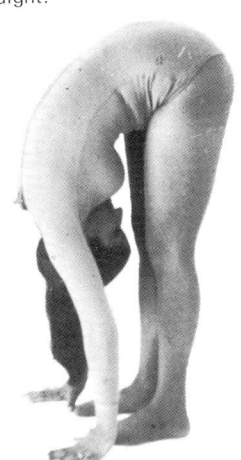

4 **Hold your breath out,** and with hands still flat on the floor, squat on your right leg and take your left leg straight back behind you.

5 Now, **inhaling,** take your right leg back so your body forms a straight line.

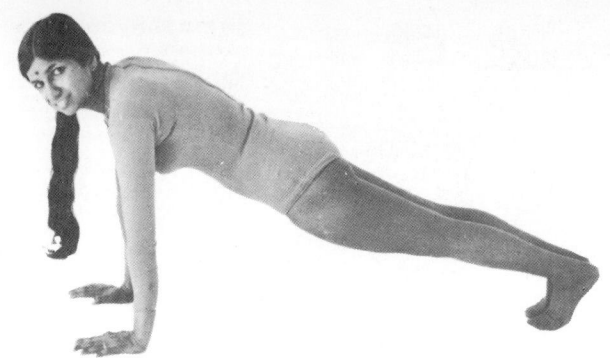

6 **Exhaling,** place your forehead, chest and knees on the ground, but be sure to keep your tummy up.

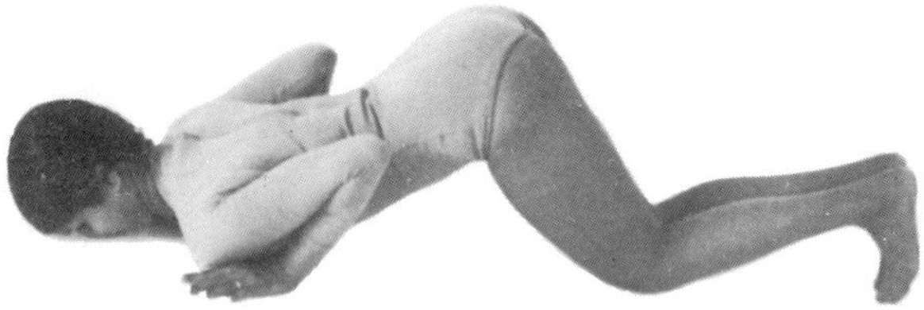

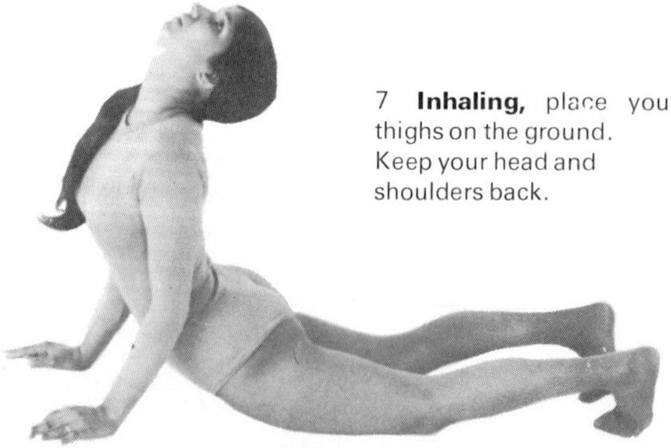

7 **Inhaling,** place your thighs on the ground. Keep your head and shoulders back.

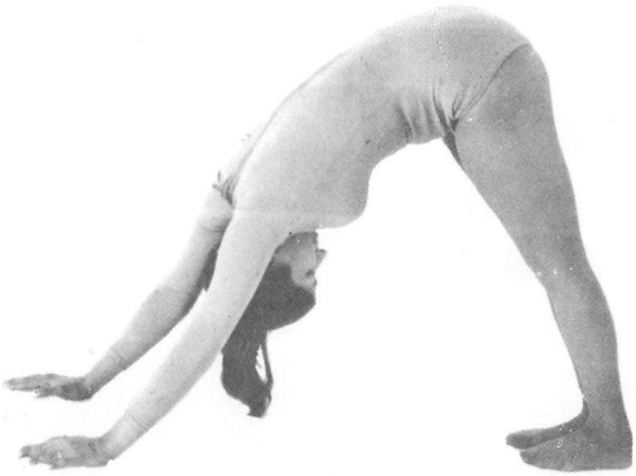

8 **Exhaling** and without moving your arms or feet, make an arch of your body.

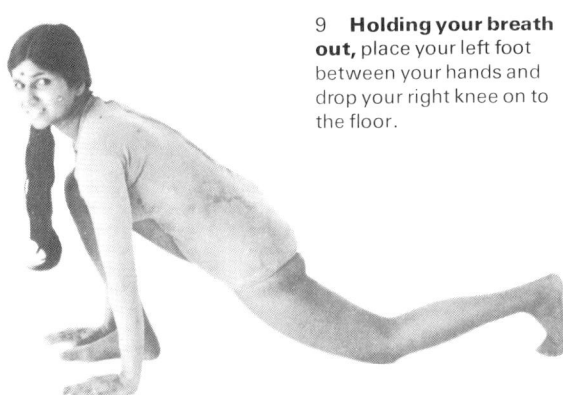

9 **Holding your breath out,** place your left foot between your hands and drop your right knee on to the floor.

10 Continue to **hold your breath out** and bring your right leg up between your hands. Straighten your knees.

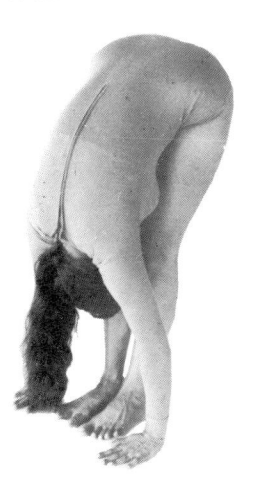

11 **Inhaling** deeply, stretch your hands above your head.

12 **Exhaling,** place your hands in prayer position in front of your chest and relax.

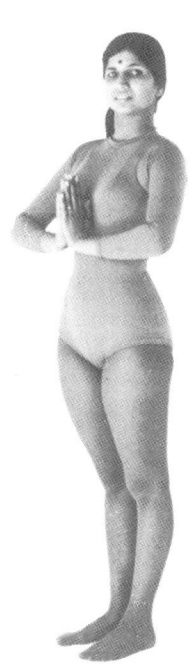

Face and Neck

Neck Circles

Neck Circles tone and firm the face and neck muscles, removing wrinkles and double chin. At the same time the tension at the back of your neck is released.

1   Slowly roll your head to the right . . .

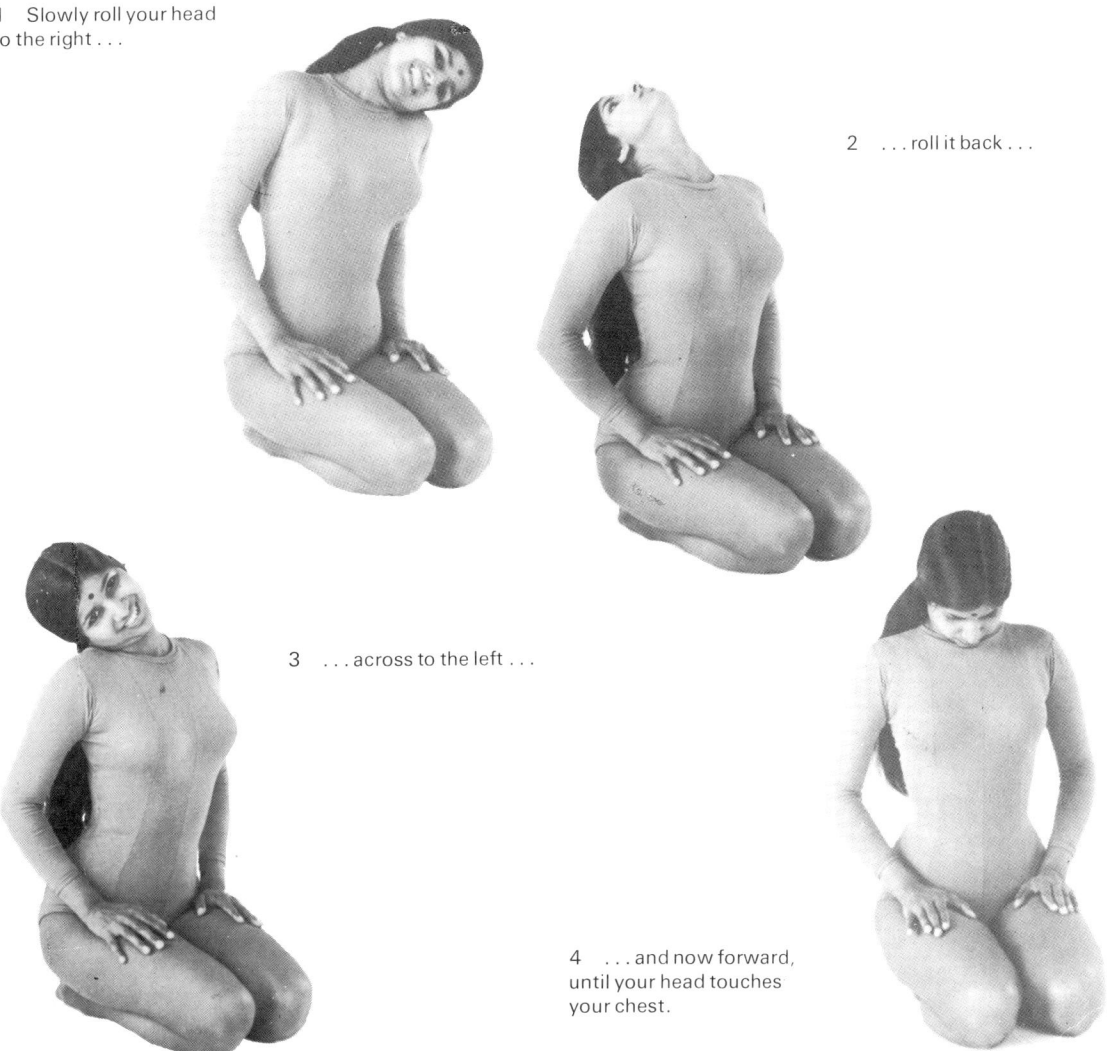

2   . . . roll it back . . .

3   . . . across to the left . . .

4   . . . and now forward, until your head touches your chest.

New Faces

No one wearing a tense, hard expression, can possibly look attractive. A few minutes spent relaxing your face each day will work wonders.

1   Puff your face as hard as you can and hold for a count of three. Relax.

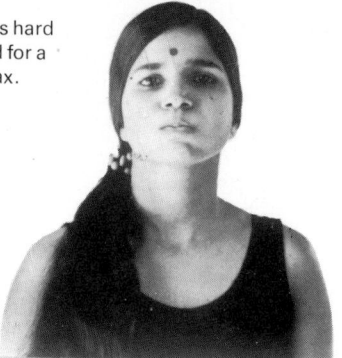

2   Puff your face and, by applying gentle pressure on your right cheek, push the air into your left cheek. Push to the right and relax.

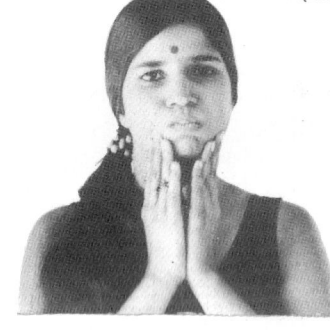

3   Suck the corners of your mouth inwards, until they join in the middle. Relax.

4   **To smooth your forehead.** Place your fingers on your forehead and draw them together and then take them apart by moving the skin beneath your fingers—**not** your fingers.

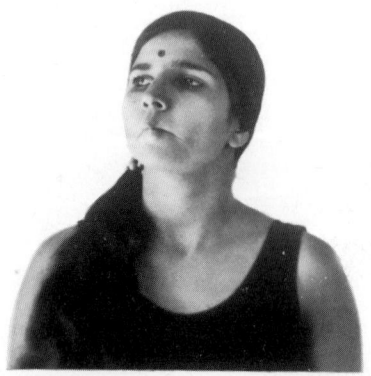

5 **Crows feet or laugh lines.** Place the back of your slightly bent index fingers on your "laugh lines" and firmly move the skin to and fro without moving your fingers.

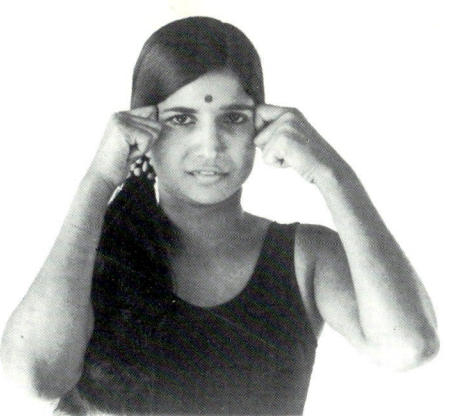

6 **Smooth your chin.** Place three fingers on your chin and move the muscles in little circles, right to left and left to right.

7 **Smooth the corners of your mouth.** Place your index fingers in the corners of your mouth, stretch and relax. Repeat three times.

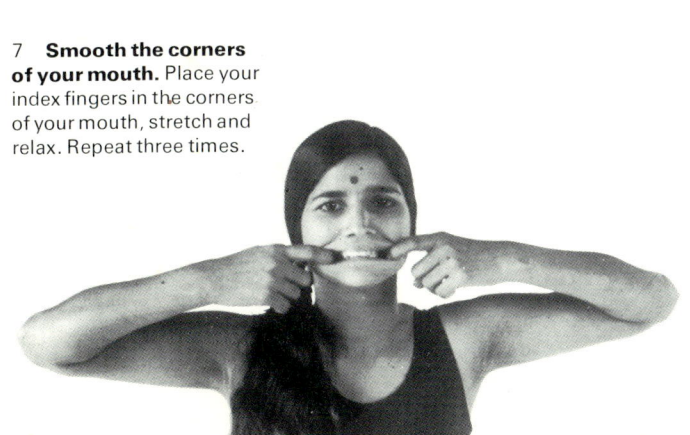

Neck Massage

To relax the tension from your face.

These exercises are more relaxing if your eyes are closed.

1   Place your fingers behind your neck, the seat of tension, and gently massage the nerves at the back of your neck.

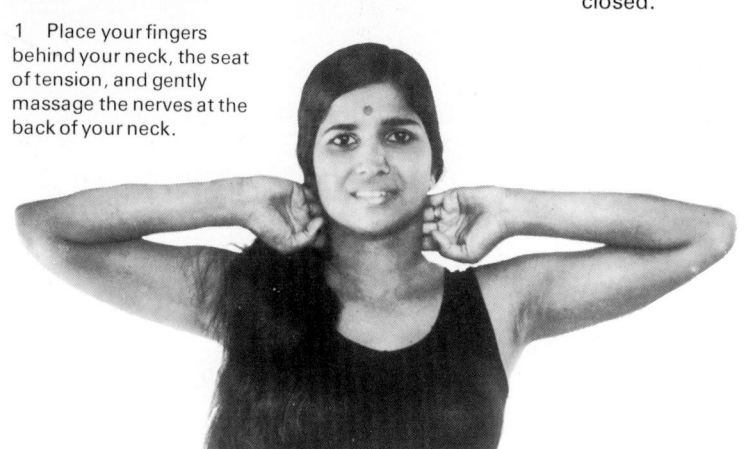

2   Fingertips on your temples, firmly massage by moving your fingers in small circles.

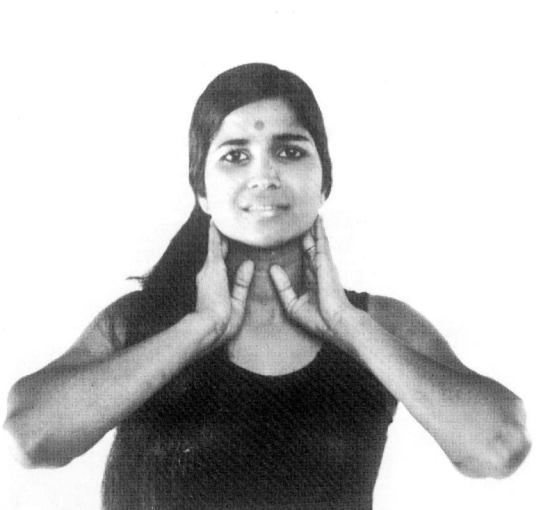

3   Now place your fingers behind your ears and massage down the sides of your neck.

Bust and Arms

Whether your bust is shapely or shapeless, flat or full, it is more attractive when carried well with your shoulders back. Mothers, don't blame your babes for your saggy bust, practised regularly, the following exercises will soon restore your firmness. They will also give small-busted girls, new confidence.

Bhujangasana (Cobra)

The beauty of your bust does not depend on the size but on its firmness and shape.
This one is marvellous for your arms as well as your bust.

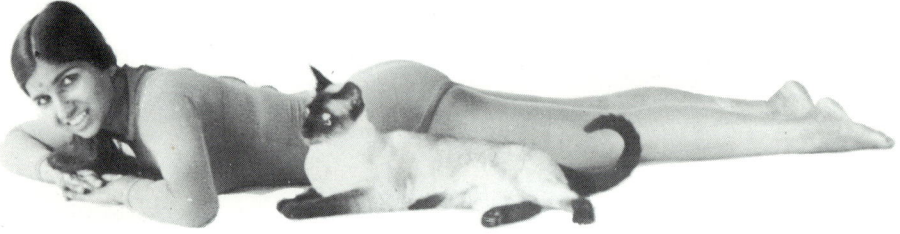

1   Lie on your tummy, fingers interlocked beneath your chin.

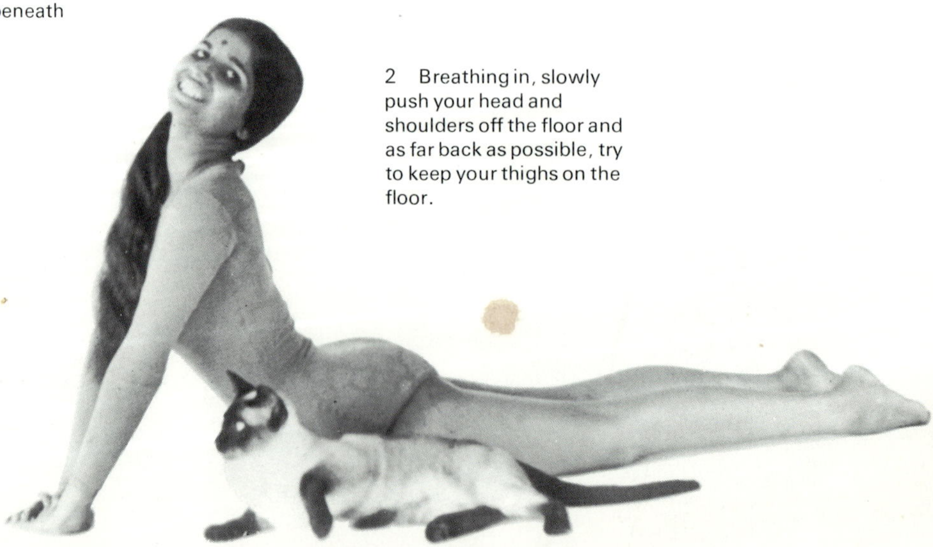

2   Breathing in, slowly push your head and shoulders off the floor and as far back as possible, try to keep your thighs on the floor.

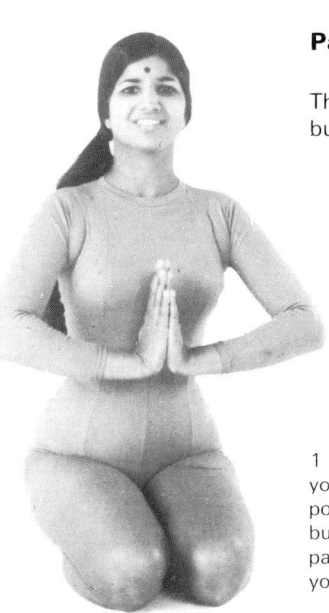

Palm Press

This exercise firms and tightens the upper arm and bust.

1   Kneel on the floor, with your hands in prayer position between your bust. Inhale and press your palms together as hard as you can. Exhale and relax.

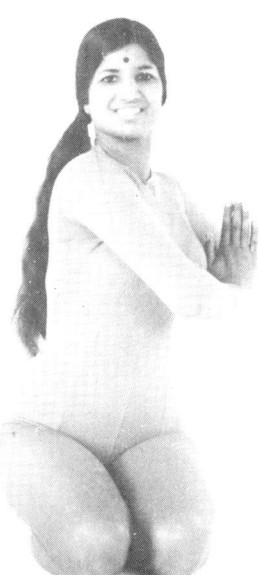

2   Repeat to the right side.

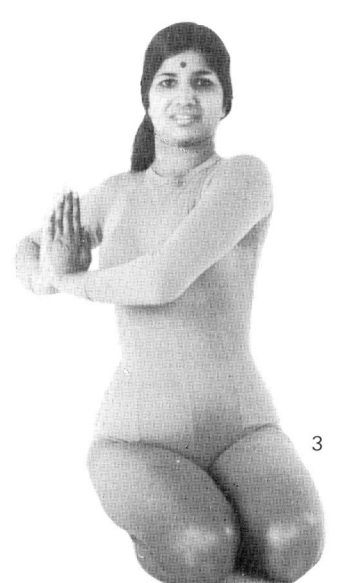

3   Now on the left side.

1 Sit on your heels, back straight, fingers interlocked behind your back, palms facing down. Inhale.

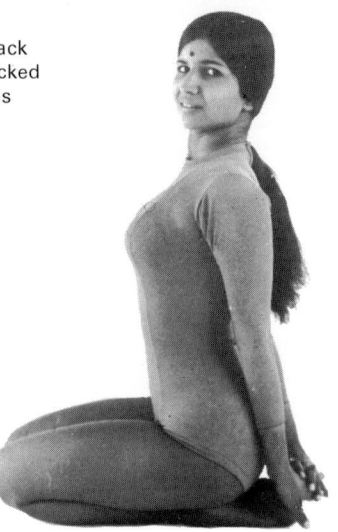

2 As you exhale, raise your hands towards your head . . .

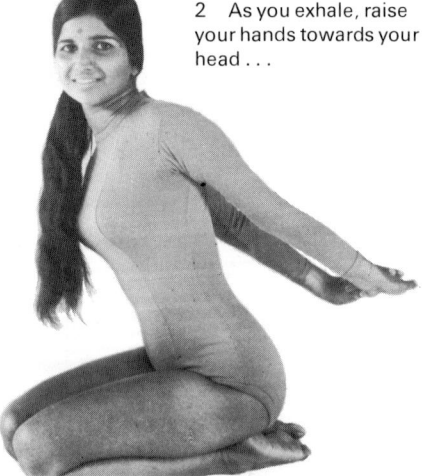

3 . . . and take your head down to the floor.

4 Breathing in, return to position 1 and relax.

Gomukhasana

Looking up to the raised elbow tones the neck muscles, uplifts your bust and firms your arms. It also exercises the seldom used muscles of your shoulders.

1 Sit in diamond posture (as shown in the photograph) with your back straight.

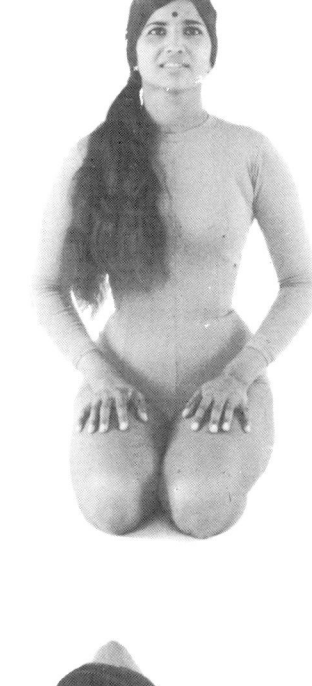

2 Take your left elbow over your left shoulder and right arm round behind your back. Clasp the fingers of both hands between your shoulder blades and look up at your raised elbow.

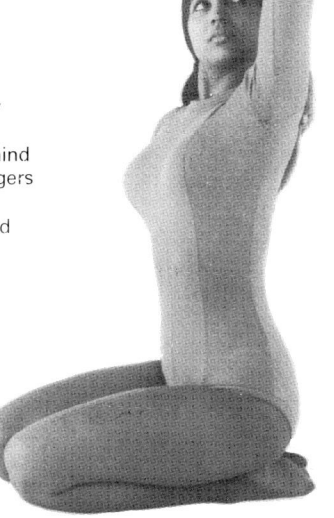

3 Repeat on the right side.

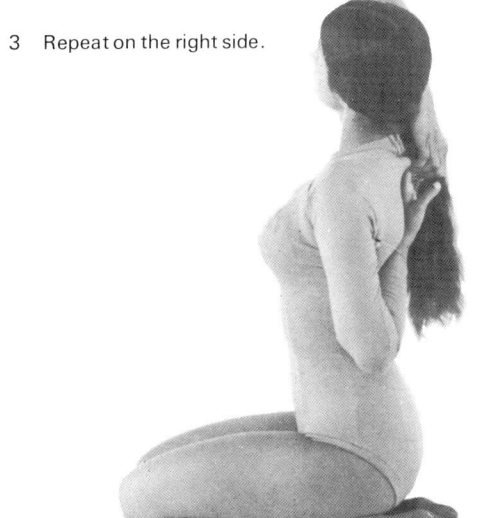

Bent Knee Push-ups

This one also tones your back.

Through yoga we become better looking, and not only improve our figure but also develop a more positive interest in life.

1   Lie on your tummy with your knees bent and your hands flat on the floor beneath your shoulders.

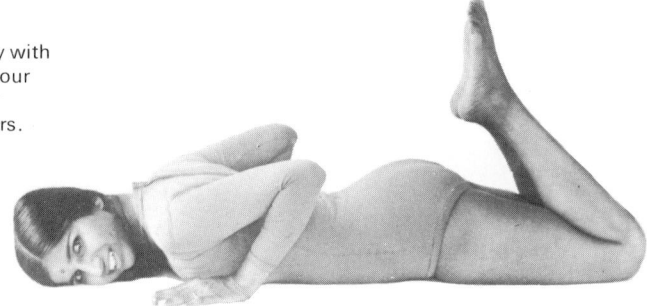

2   Inhaling, slowly push yourself up on your arms, keeping your knees bent.

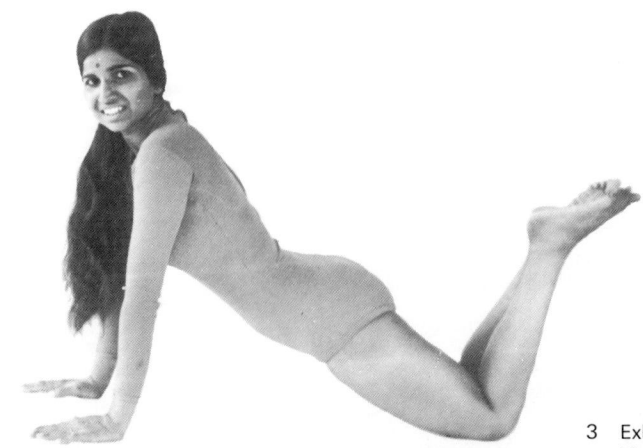

3   Exhaling, return to position 1. Repeat three times and relax.

To Improve Your Posture
as well as Your Bust

1   Kneel on the floor with your fingers interlocked behind your neck.

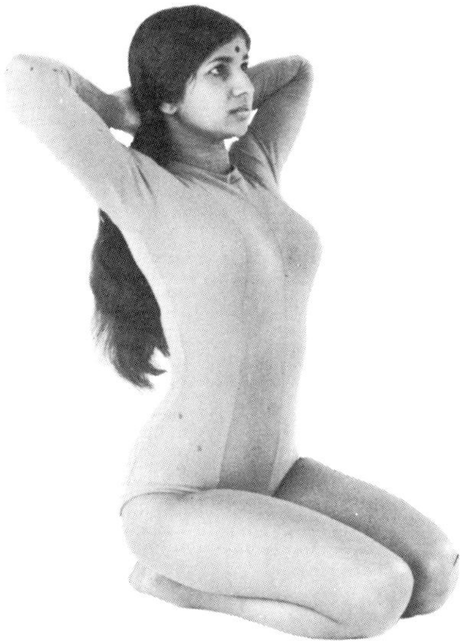

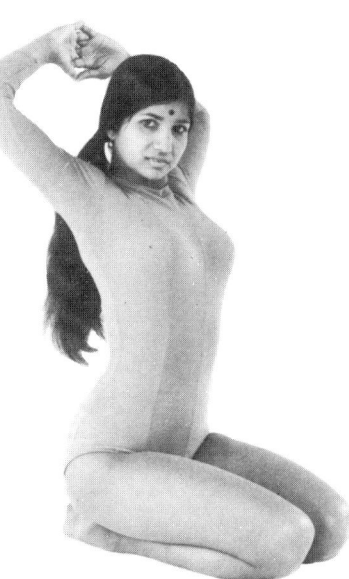

2   Inhaling deeply, raise your hands up and back . . .

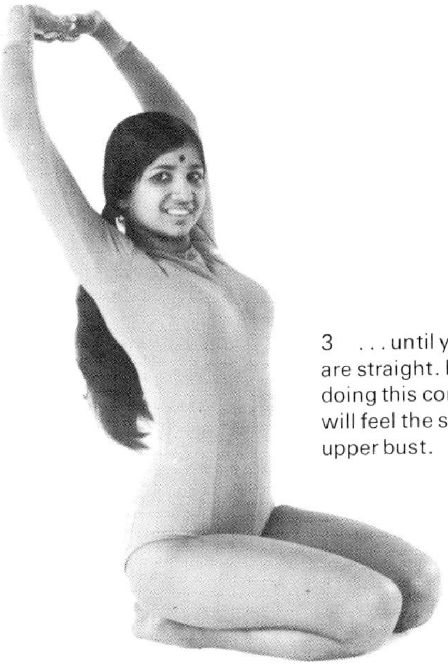

3   . . . until your elbows are straight. If you are doing this correctly, you will feel the stretch on the upper bust.

33

Side Push-ups

Especially for your arms.

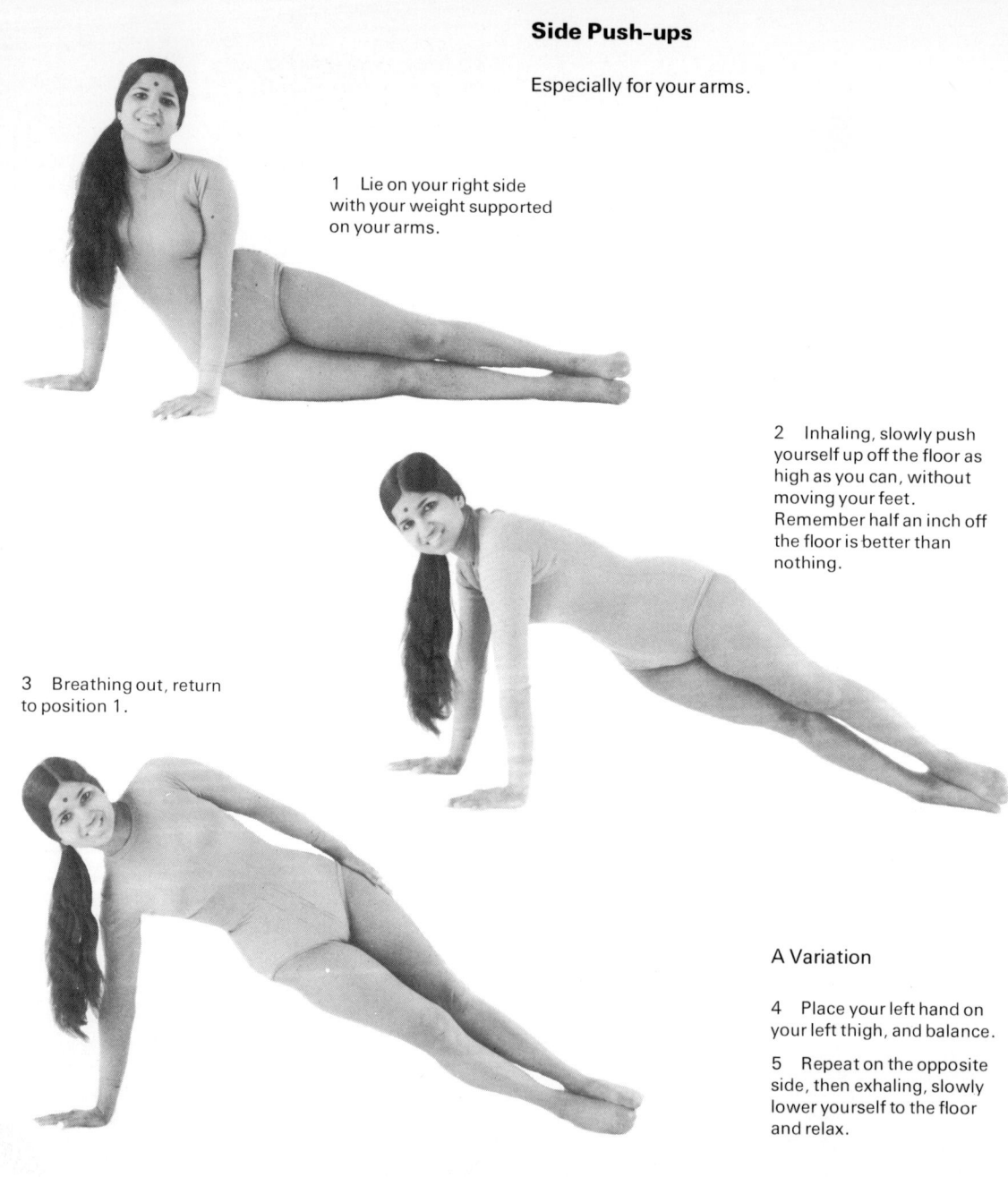

1 Lie on your right side with your weight supported on your arms.

2 Inhaling, slowly push yourself up off the floor as high as you can, without moving your feet. Remember half an inch off the floor is better than nothing.

3 Breathing out, return to position 1.

A Variation

4 Place your left hand on your left thigh, and balance.

5 Repeat on the opposite side, then exhaling, slowly lower yourself to the floor and relax.

Tummy and Waist

Tummy

A flat tummy not only looks trim but means that your internal organs are being held in place too. But remember, just as it has taken some years to gain your excess weight, you are not going to become slim overnight.

Halasana (Plough)

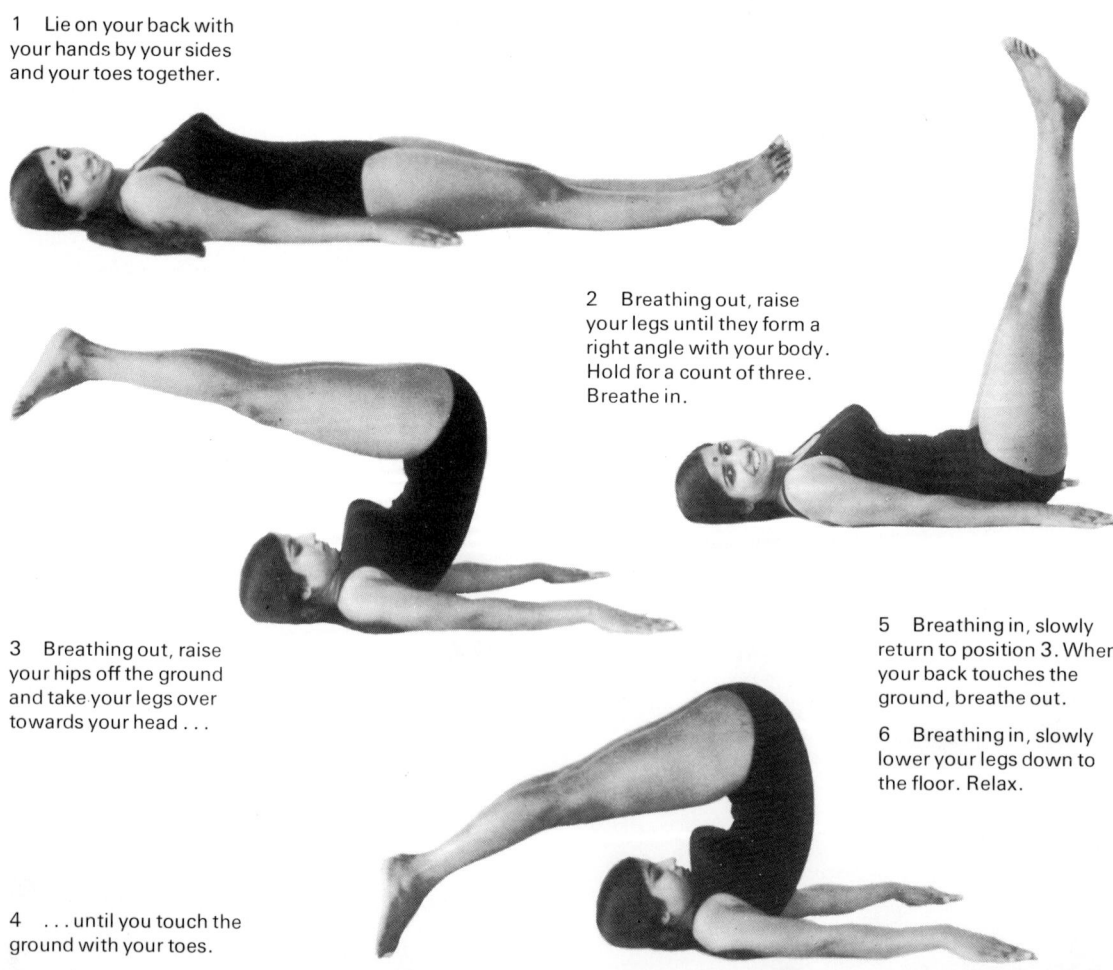

1   Lie on your back with your hands by your sides and your toes together.

2   Breathing out, raise your legs until they form a right angle with your body. Hold for a count of three. Breathe in.

3   Breathing out, raise your hips off the ground and take your legs over towards your head . . .

4   . . . until you touch the ground with your toes.

5   Breathing in, slowly return to position 3. When your back touches the ground, breathe out.

6   Breathing in, slowly lower your legs down to the floor. Relax.

Cross-Overs

Beginners. Practise as many cross-overs as you can raising your legs as high as possible.

1   Support yourself on your elbows in half reclining position and raise your legs, at the same time crossing your left foot over your right.

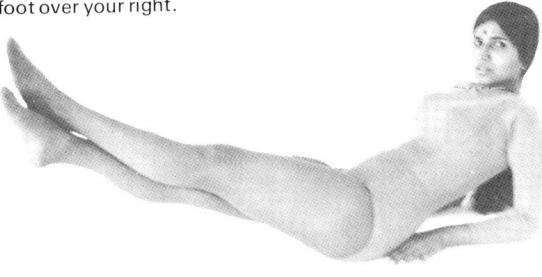

2   Then right over left.

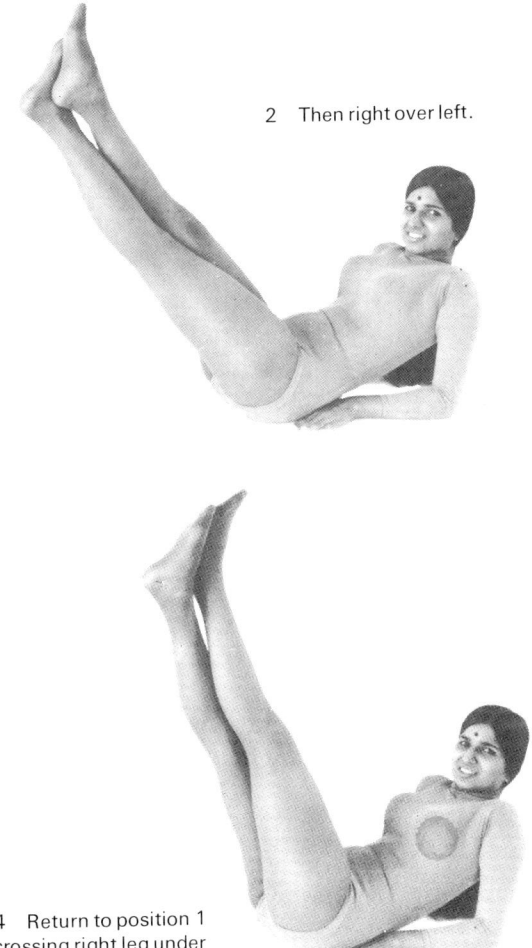

3   Left over right again. Your legs should now be perpendicular with the floor.

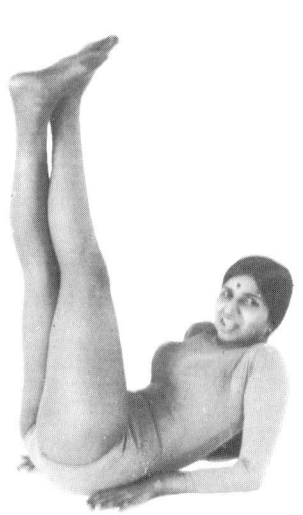

4   Return to position 1 crossing right leg under left etc.

Toe Touching

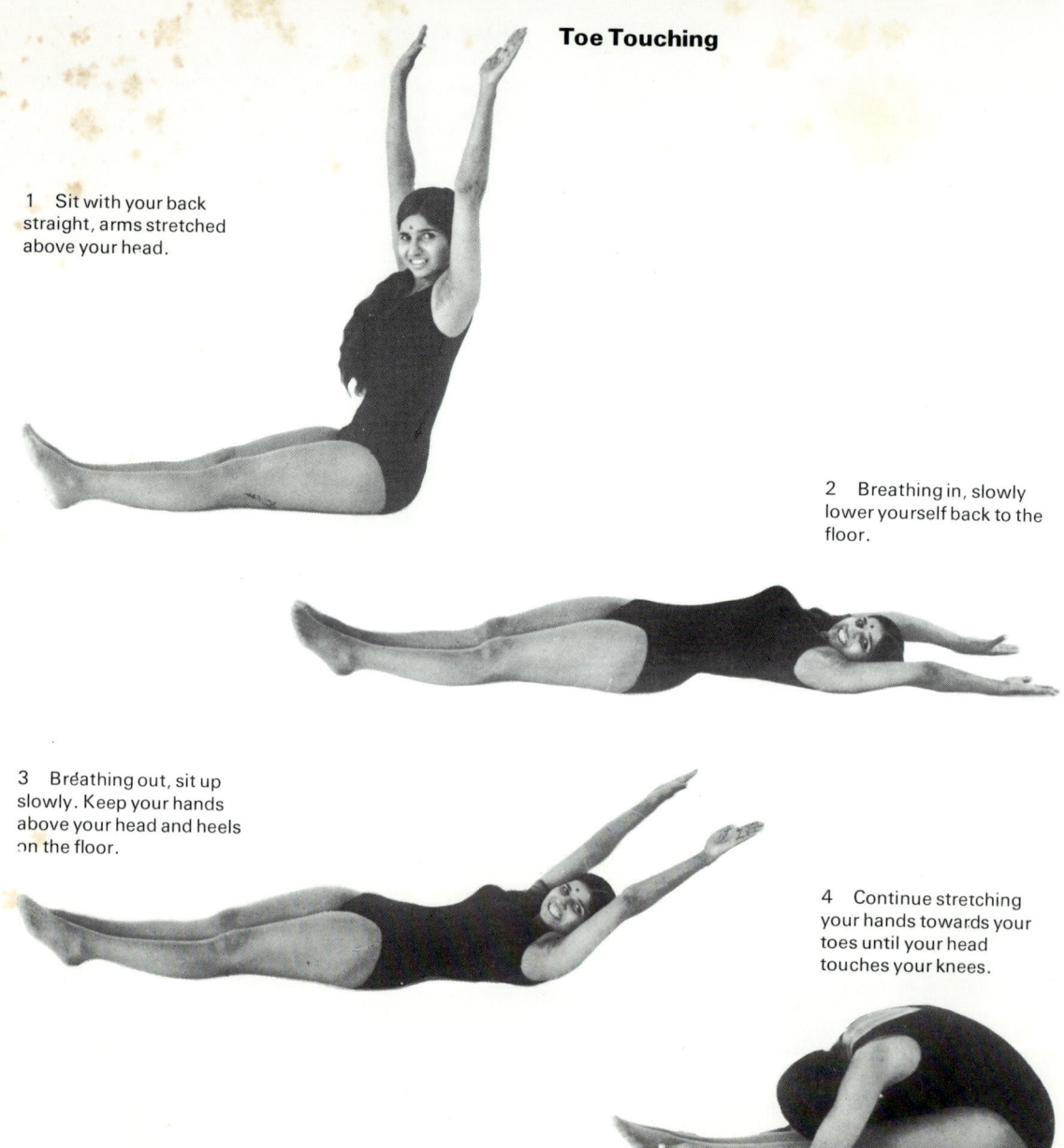

1 Sit with your back straight, arms stretched above your head.

2 Breathing in, slowly lower yourself back to the floor.

3 Breathing out, sit up slowly. Keep your hands above your head and heels on the floor.

4 Continue stretching your hands towards your toes until your head touches your knees.

Waist

It is easier to be wise for others, than to be wise for ourselves. It is easy for us to see what others should do to stay young, to lose weight and to slim their waist, but there is an old Indian saying, "The easiest way to get anything is to earn it," and this applies to trimming your waist.

Trikonasana

1   Stand with your feet wide apart, and arms outstretched at shoulder level.

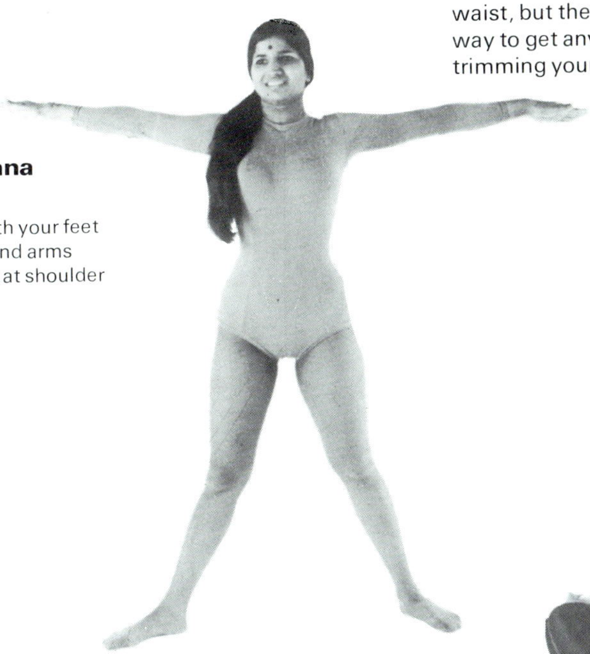

2   Breathing out, twist to the right side, taking your left hand across to your right foot. Look up at the back of your right hand.

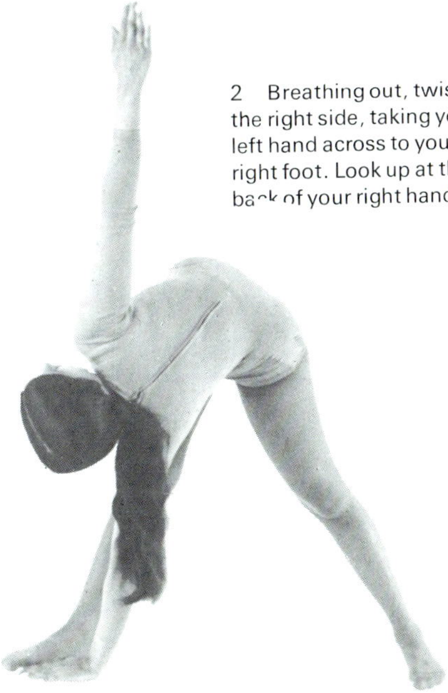

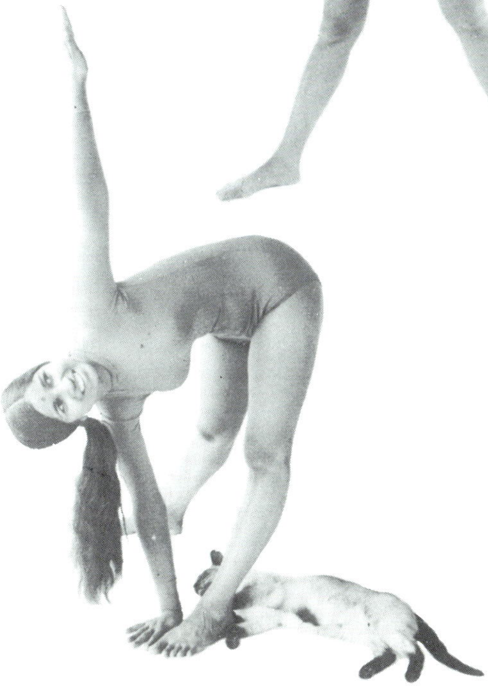

3   Repeat on the opposite side. Make sure you keep your knees straight.

Standing Waist Sway

A simple but successful waist trimmer.

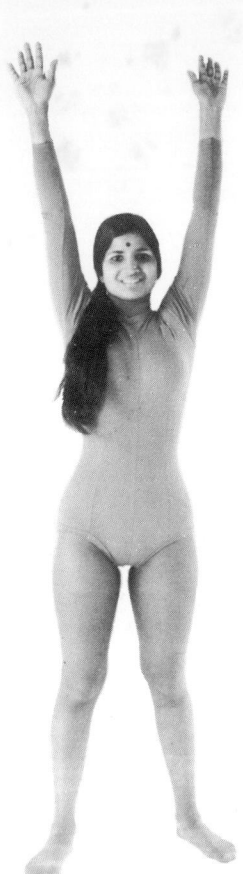

1 Feet slightly apart to give you balance, inhale and stretch your hands over your head.

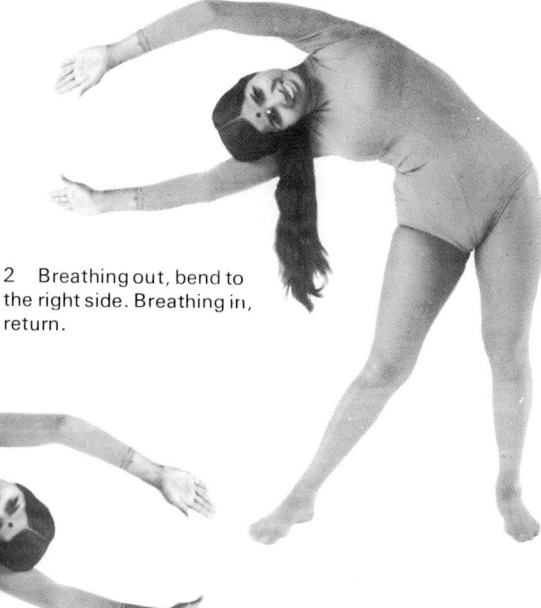

2 Breathing out, bend to the right side. Breathing in, return.

3 Breathing out, bend to the left. Inhaling, return and relax.

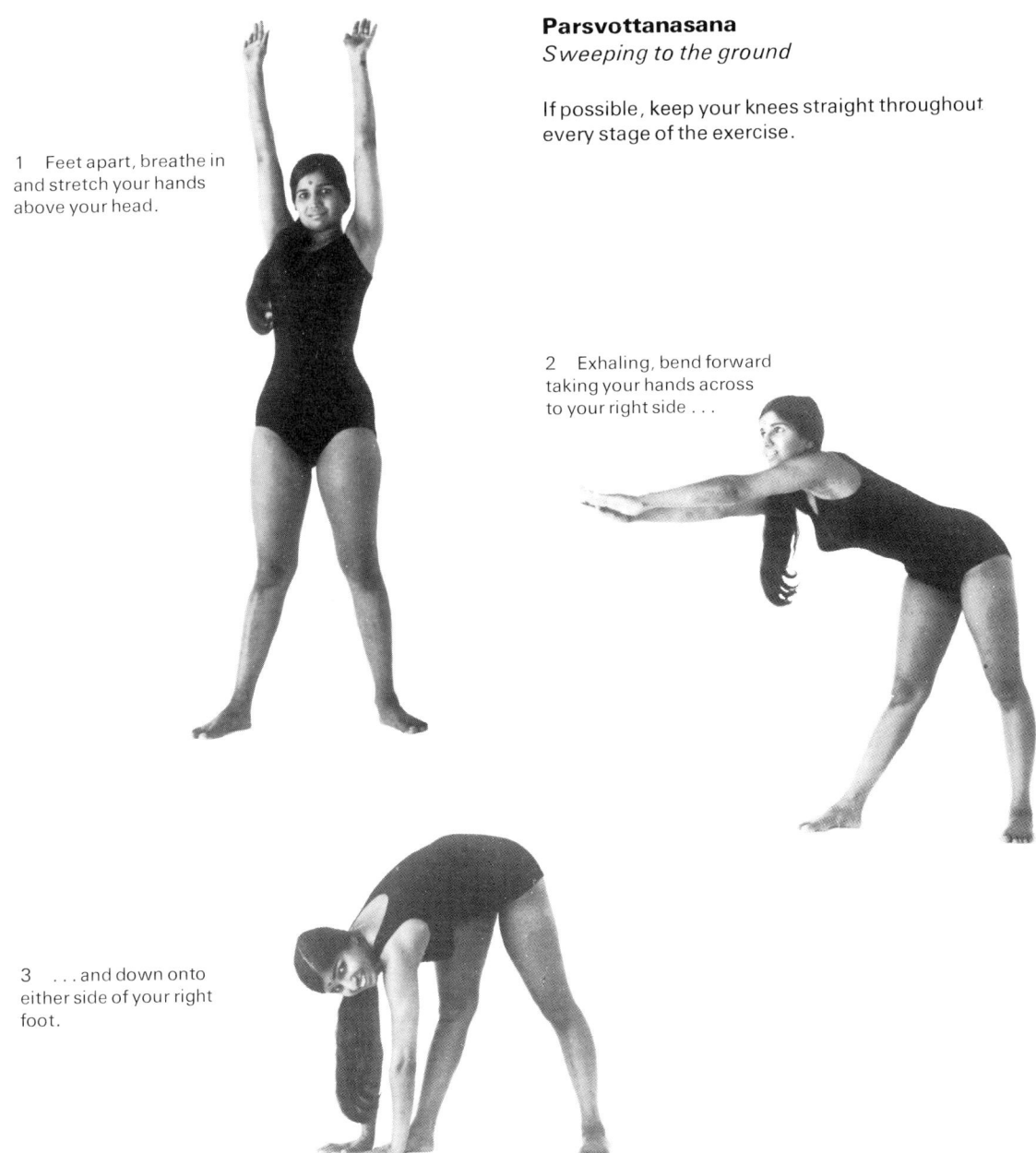

Parsvottanasana
Sweeping to the ground

If possible, keep your knees straight throughout every stage of the exercise.

1 Feet apart, breathe in and stretch your hands above your head.

2 Exhaling, bend forward taking your hands across to your right side . . .

3 . . . and down onto either side of your right foot.

4 Slide your hands across to your left foot.

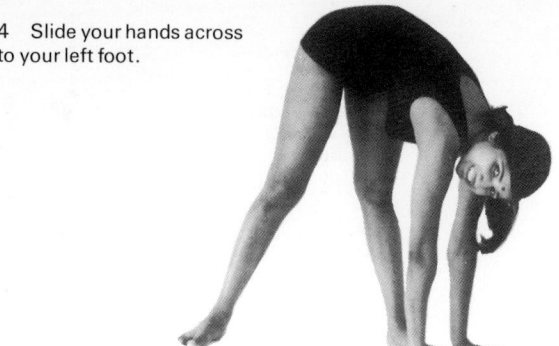

5 Inhaling, slowly return to position 1, exhaling, lower your hands.

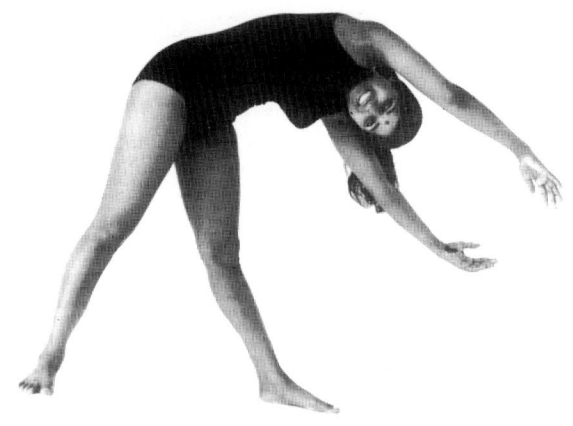

6 Repeat on the other side.

Hips

We all know that daily exercise and sensible eating are necessary to maintain good health but how many of us really try to practise this? Either through misuse of time, or mistaken values we neglect our health and appearance, and because we grow too fat for fashions are forced to wear any old thing.

The Hip Trimmer

This removes unsightly bulges and lumps.

1   Support yourself on your elbows with your knees bent.

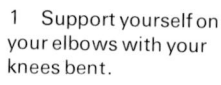

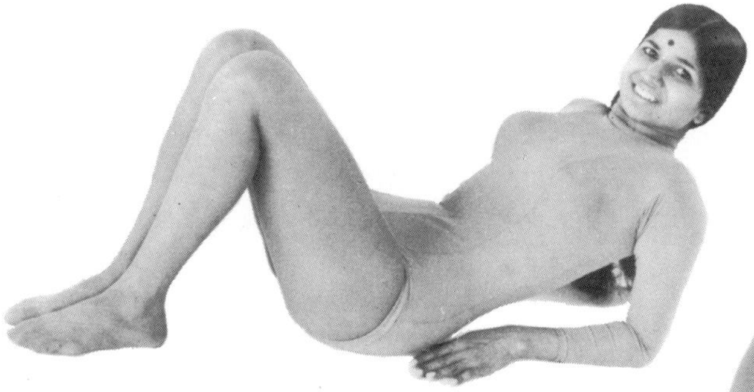

2   Exhaling, take your knees to the right side, without lifting your elbows off the ground. Inhaling, return.

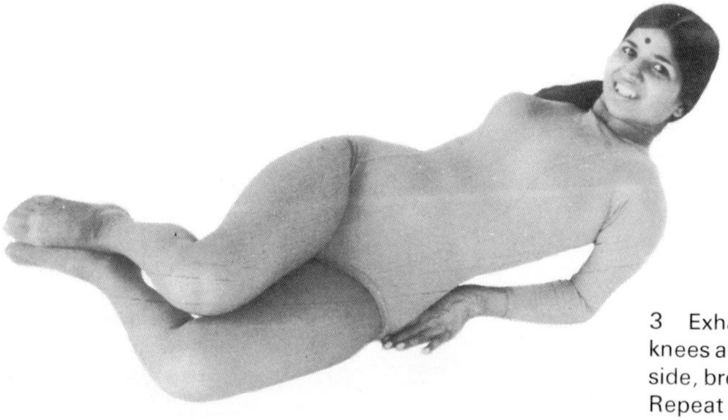

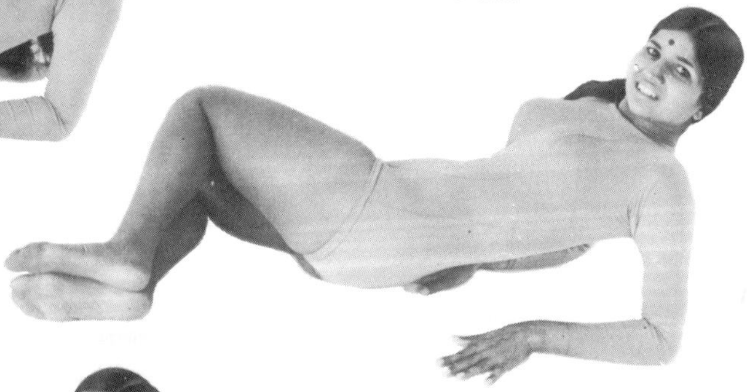

3   Exhaling, take your knees across to the left side, breathing in return. Repeat twice and relax.

Forward Lunge

Also recommended for pregnant women.

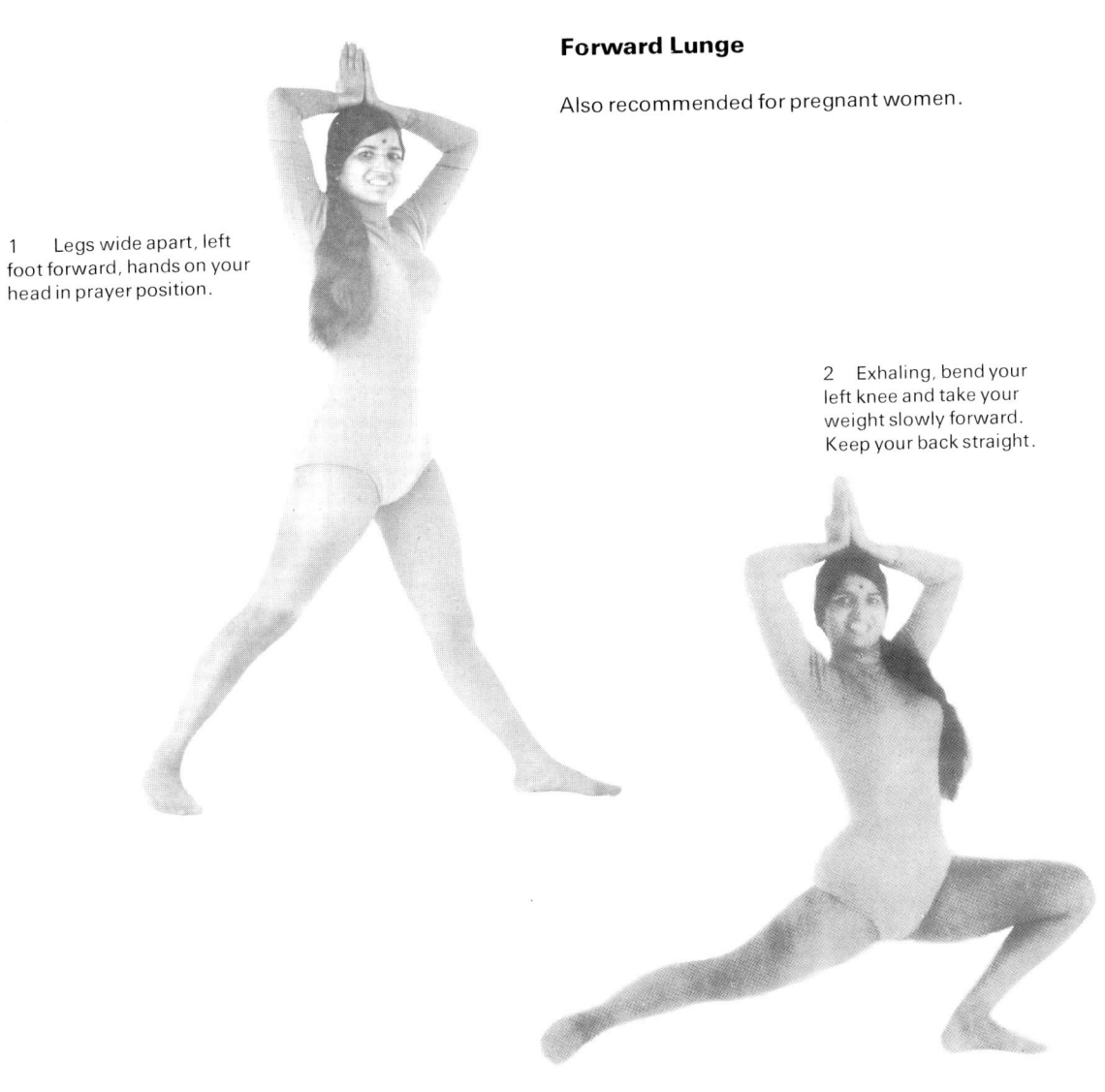

1 Legs wide apart, left foot forward, hands on your head in prayer position.

2 Exhaling, bend your left knee and take your weight slowly forward. Keep your back straight.

3 Inhaling, slowly return to position 1 and repeat on the other side.

Akarna-Dhanurasana (Archer)

This reduces your hips and gives you determination and concentration.

1   Breathing in, grasp your left foot (which should be resting across your right thigh) with your right hand, and touch your right toes with your left hand.

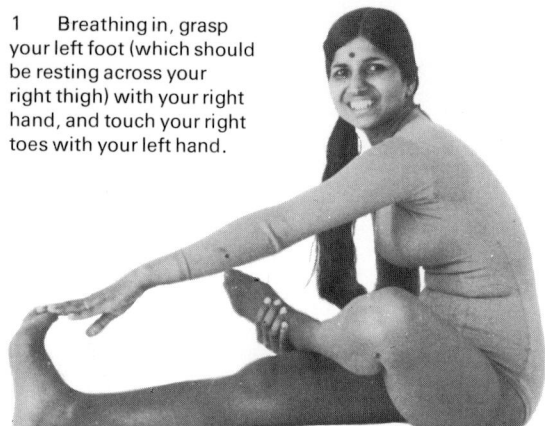

2 .Exhaling, raise your left foot to your right ear.

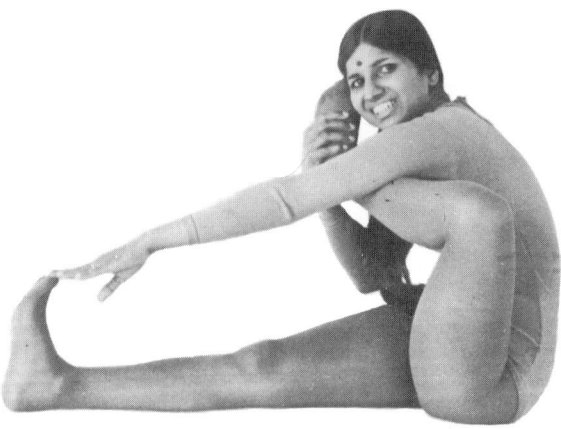

3   Breathing in, return to position 1, and repeat on the other side.

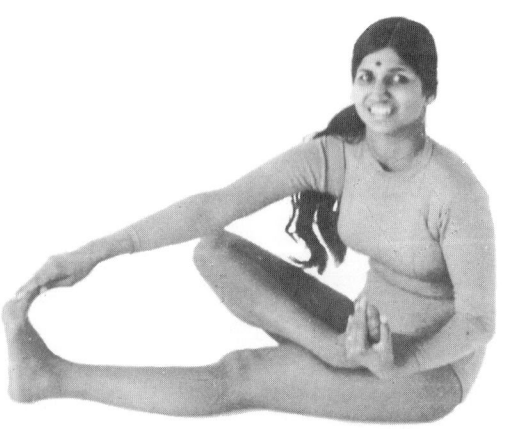

Hip Pointer

This massages the pubic region and lower back.

1   Lie on your left side, supporting yourself on your left elbow.

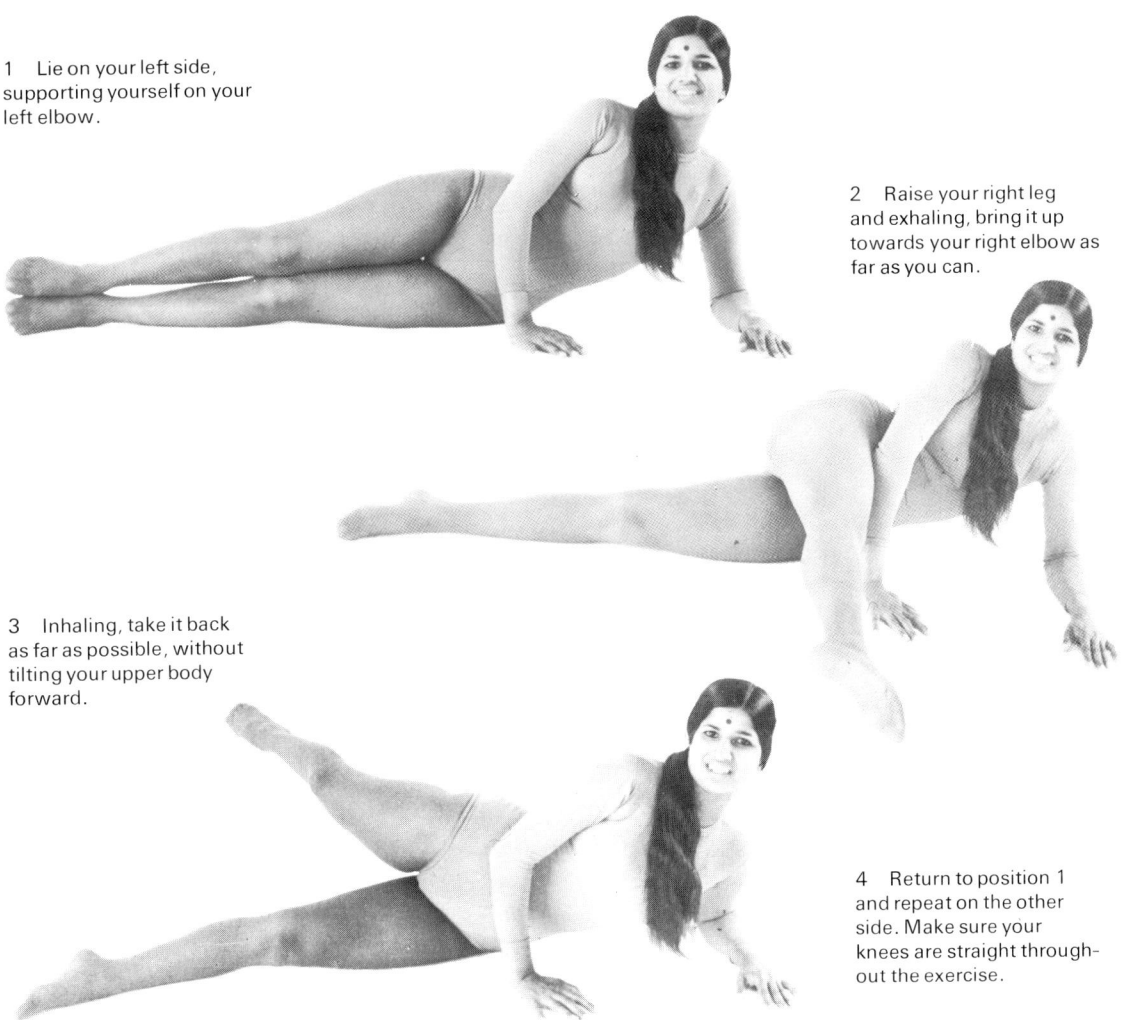

2   Raise your right leg and exhaling, bring it up towards your right elbow as far as you can.

3   Inhaling, take it back as far as possible, without tilting your upper body forward.

4   Return to position 1 and repeat on the other side. Make sure your knees are straight throughout the exercise.

Ardha Chandrasana (The Crescent Moon)

This asana is good for your in-steps, ankles, calf muscles and inner thighs. It also reduces your waist and hips.

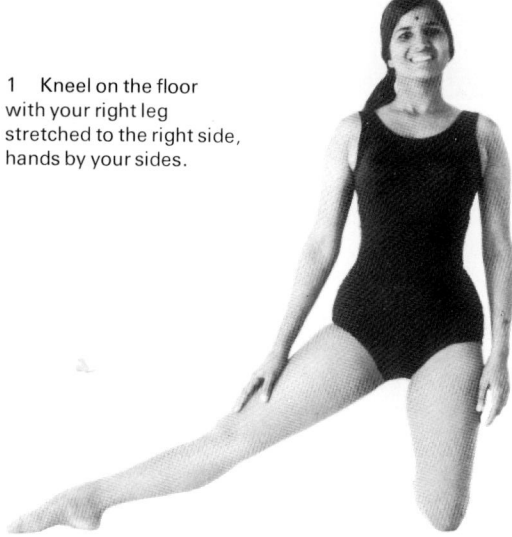

1 Kneel on the floor with your right leg stretched to the right side, hands by your sides.

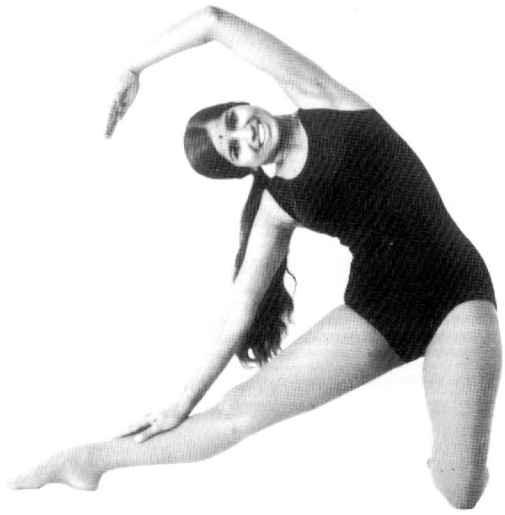

2 Exhaling, slide your right hand towards your right ankle and stretch your left hand above your head.

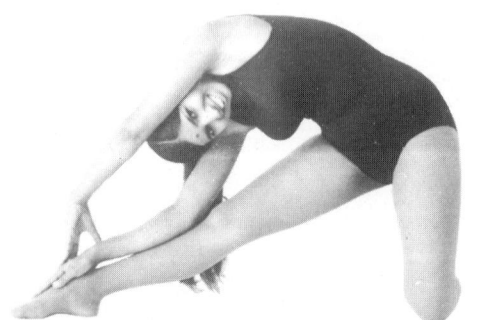

3 Try to place your left hand on top of your right hand, without bending forward.

Hippy Magic

Although a little difficult, this exercise does wonders to your hips.
It also helps prevent arthritis of your hip and firms your buttocks and thighs.

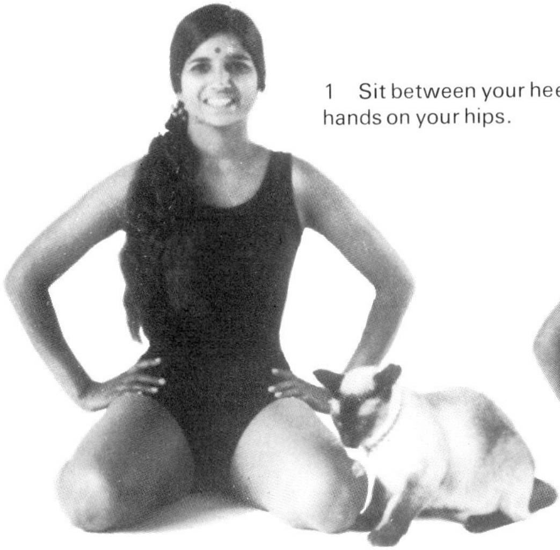

1 Sit between your heels, hands on your hips.

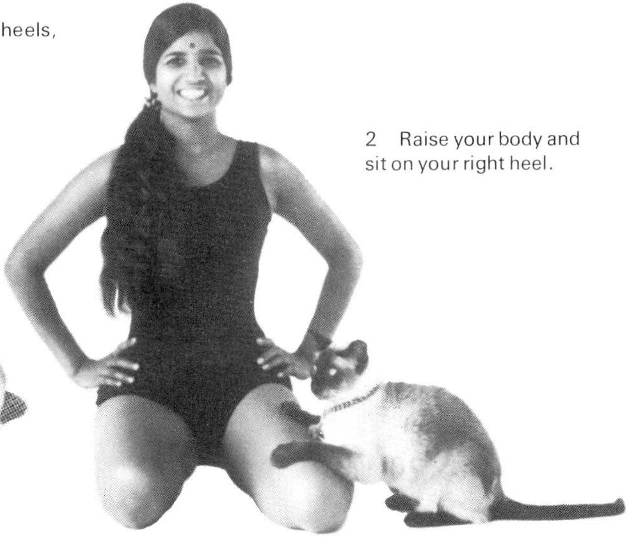

2 Raise your body and sit on your right heel.

3 Lifting your left leg bring it forward and place your left foot flat on the floor in line with your right knee.

4 Now sit between your heels.

5 Return step by step to position 1 and repeat with the other leg.

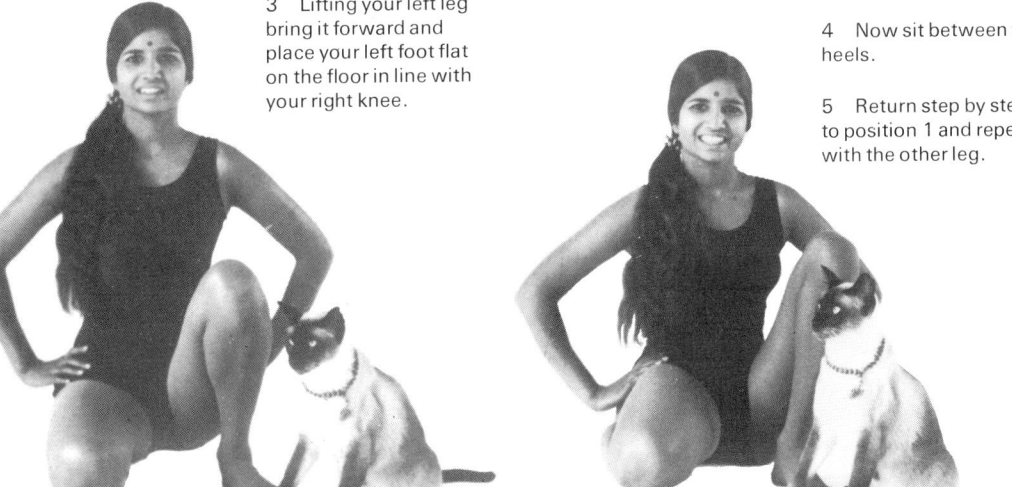

Sacro-Sway

This asana reduces your waist, hips and thighs.

1   Sit in diamond posture, fingers interlocked on your thighs.

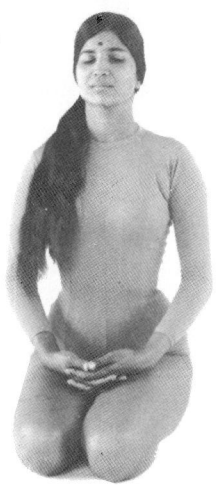

2   Inhaling, raise yourself up off your heels, taking your hands high above your head at the same time.

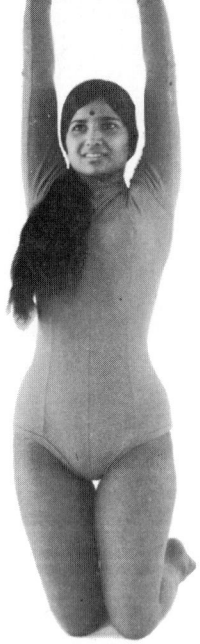

3   Exhaling, sit on your right side. Inhaling, return to the second position.

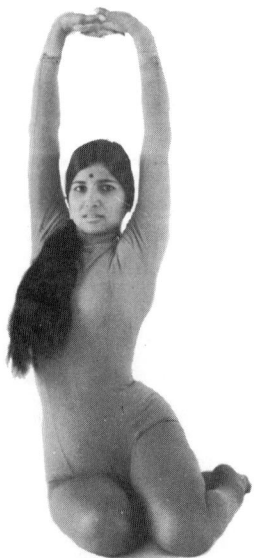

5   Exhaling, sit on your left side. Inhaling, slowly return to second position, then exhaling slowly, return to position 1.

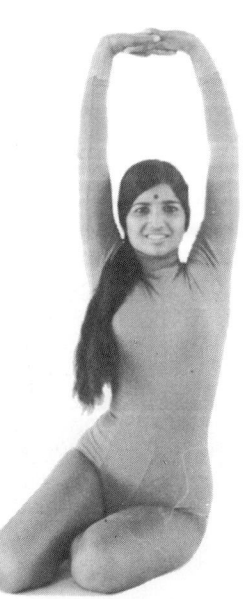

Thighs

God, help me to blame myself if my thighs are fat. I am the only one who can exercise, no one can do it for me. Yoga exercise is not for the young, yoga is the means of staying young.

1   Stand on your toes, right leg in front of your left, hands on your waist.

One Leg Squat

To shape your ankles, legs and thighs

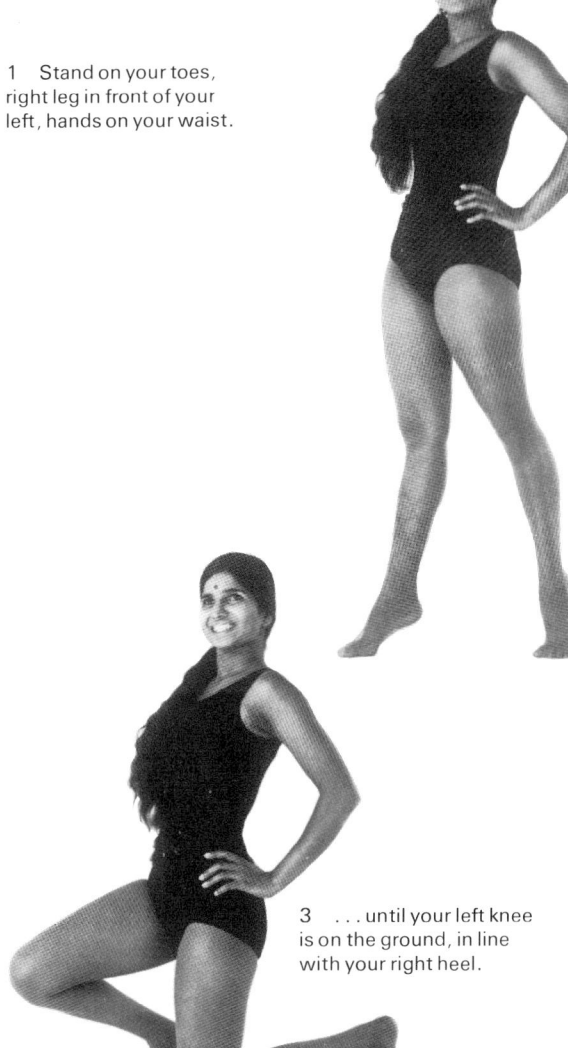

2   Breathing out, slowly lower yourself down to the floor (keeping your back straight) . . .

3   . . . until your left knee is on the ground, in line with your right heel.

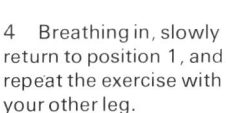

4   Breathing in, slowly return to position 1, and repeat the exercise with your other leg.

51

Extreme Stretch

1   Sit with your knees bent, hands firmly on the ground.

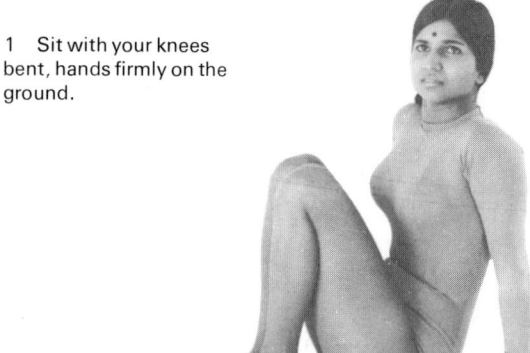

2   Slowly push yourself up on your toes, until you are sitting on your heels.

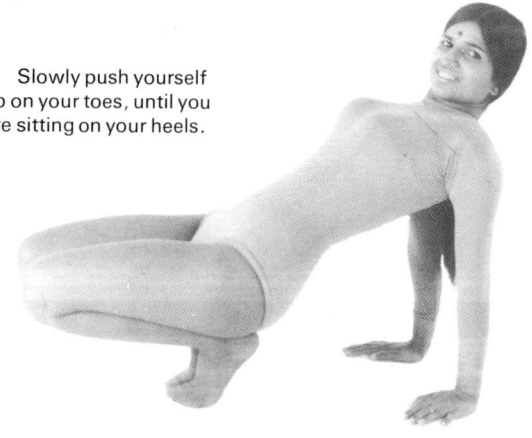

3   Without moving your hands, drop your knees to the ground, and drop your head back.

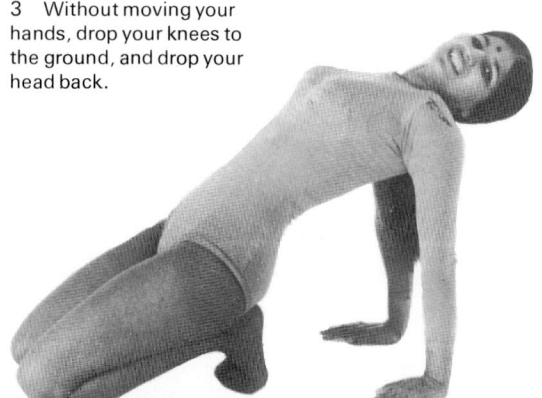

4   Breathing out, bring your head forward and slowly return to position 1. Relax.

Suptavajrasana
Lying flat in diamond posture

1   Sit between your feet with your hands on the soles of your feet.

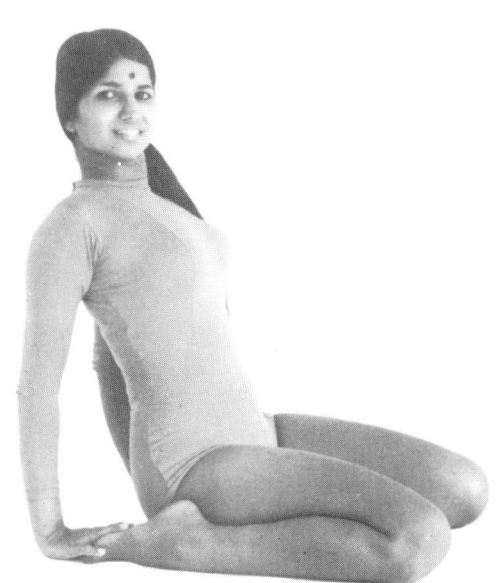

2   Breathing in and slowly bending your elbows, lower yourself to the ground. Try to keep your knees on the ground and don't move your hands.

3   Slowly lift your shoulders off the ground by arching your back. Place your hands in prayer position in front of your chest.

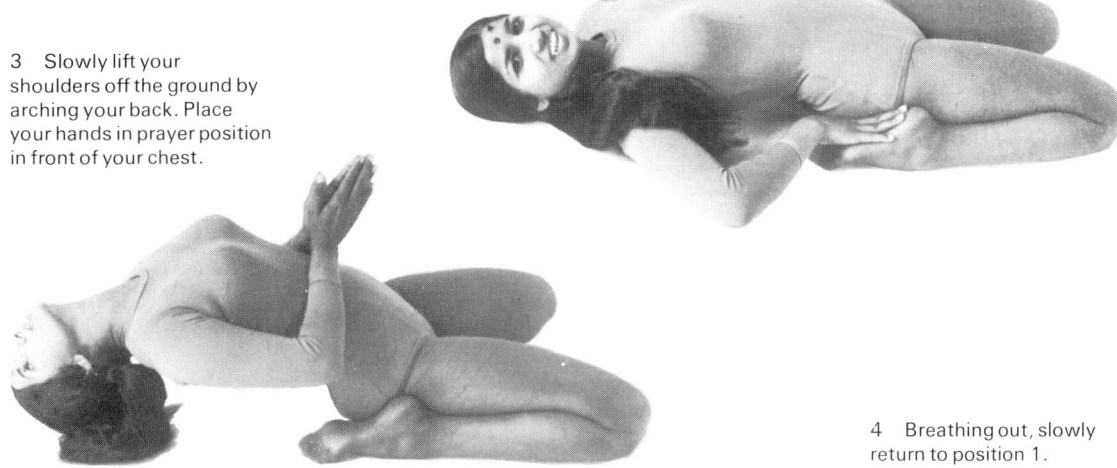

4   Breathing out, slowly return to position 1.

Legs

To Shape the Legs

All women dream of beautiful legs, but it will remain a dream until we get them moving.

1   With your hands on your hips, and weight on your right leg, swing your left leg across to the right.

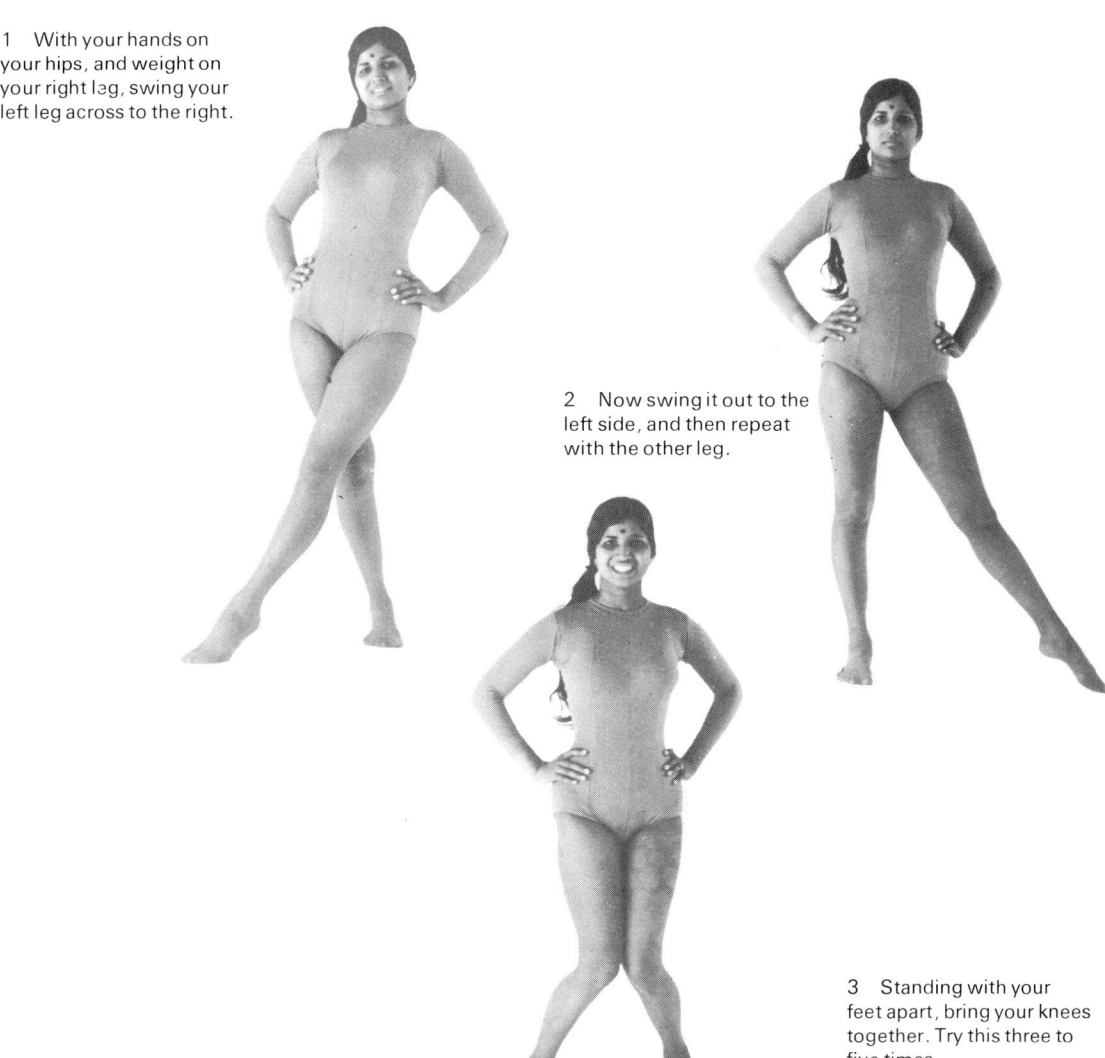

2   Now swing it out to the left side, and then repeat with the other leg.

3   Standing with your feet apart, bring your knees together. Try this three to five times.

Anantasana
Side Leg-Raise

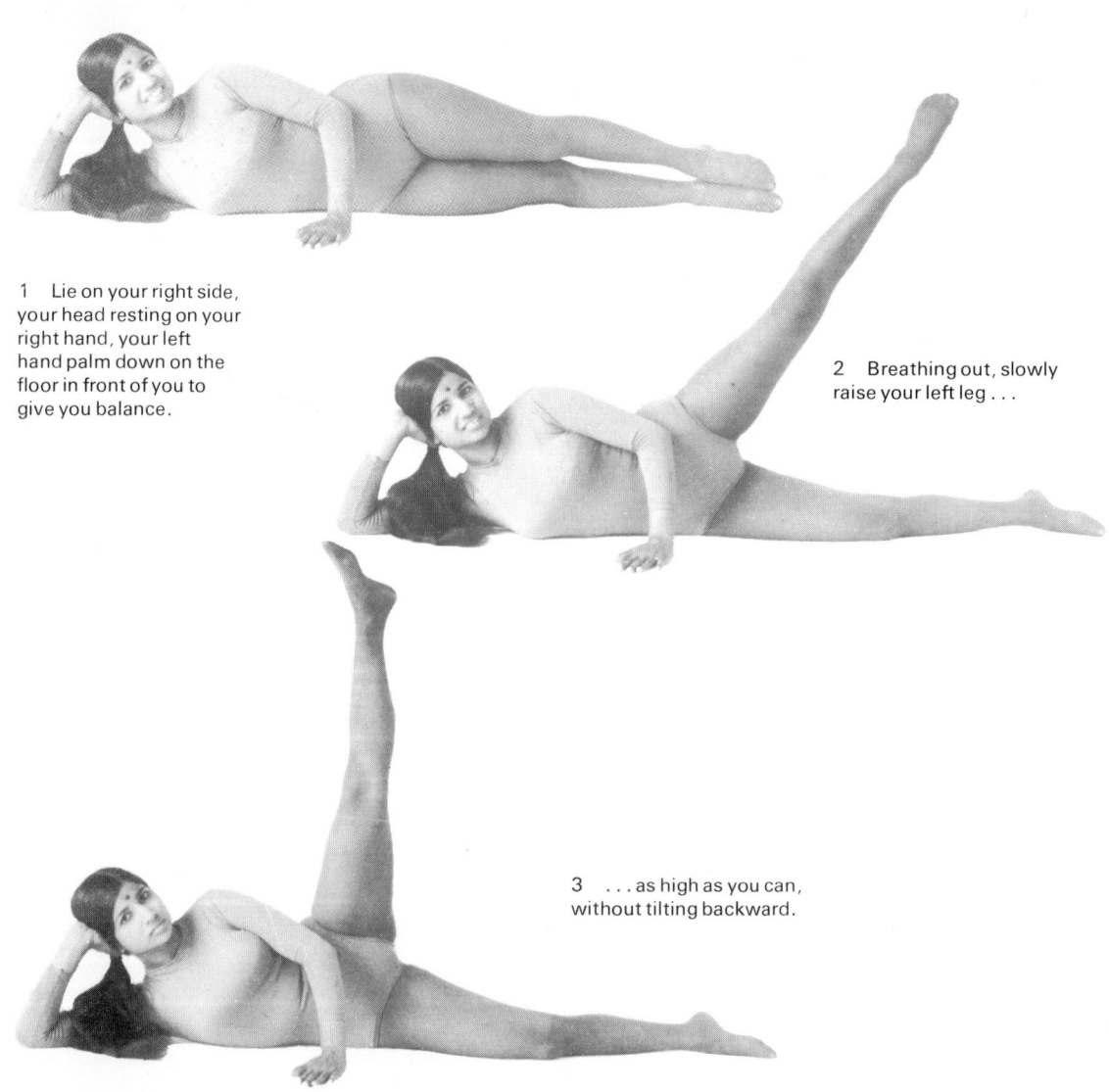

1   Lie on your right side, your head resting on your right hand, your left hand palm down on the floor in front of you to give you balance.

2   Breathing out, slowly raise your left leg . . .

3   . . . as high as you can, without tilting backward.

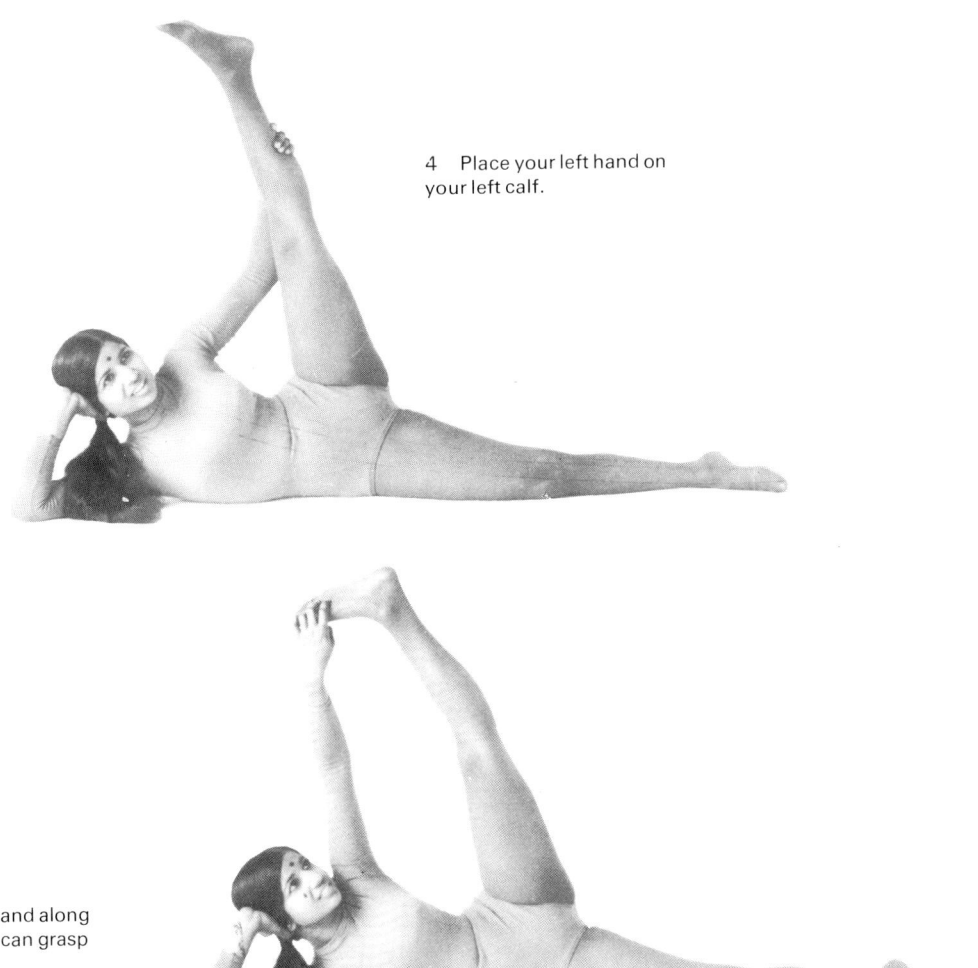

4   Place your left hand on
your left calf.

5   Slide your hand along
your leg till you can grasp
your left toes.

6   Slowly return to position
1 and repeat with your
right leg.

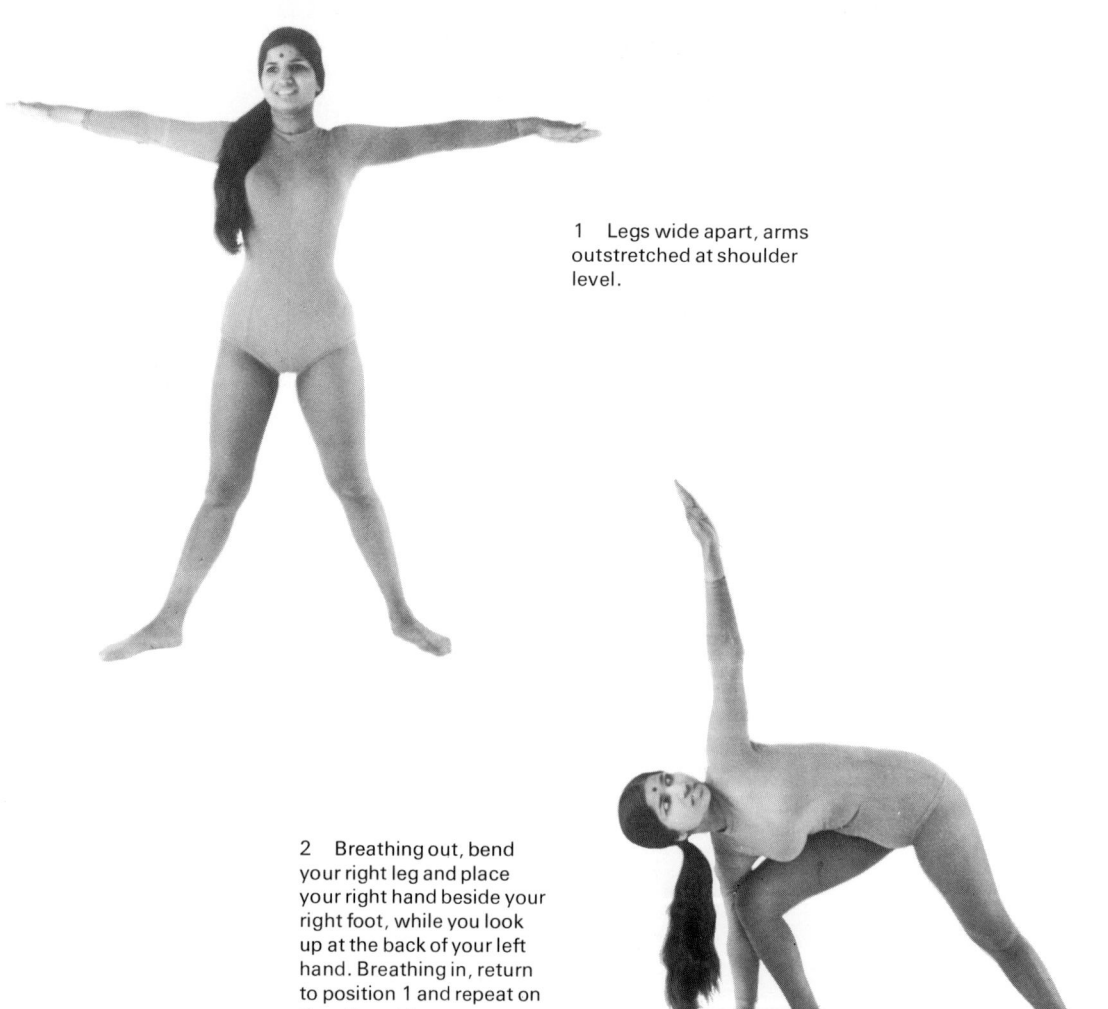

1 Legs wide apart, arms outstretched at shoulder level.

2 Breathing out, bend your right leg and place your right hand beside your right foot, while you look up at the back of your left hand. Breathing in, return to position 1 and repeat on the other side.

The Leg Stretch

This puts a spring in your step whatever your age.

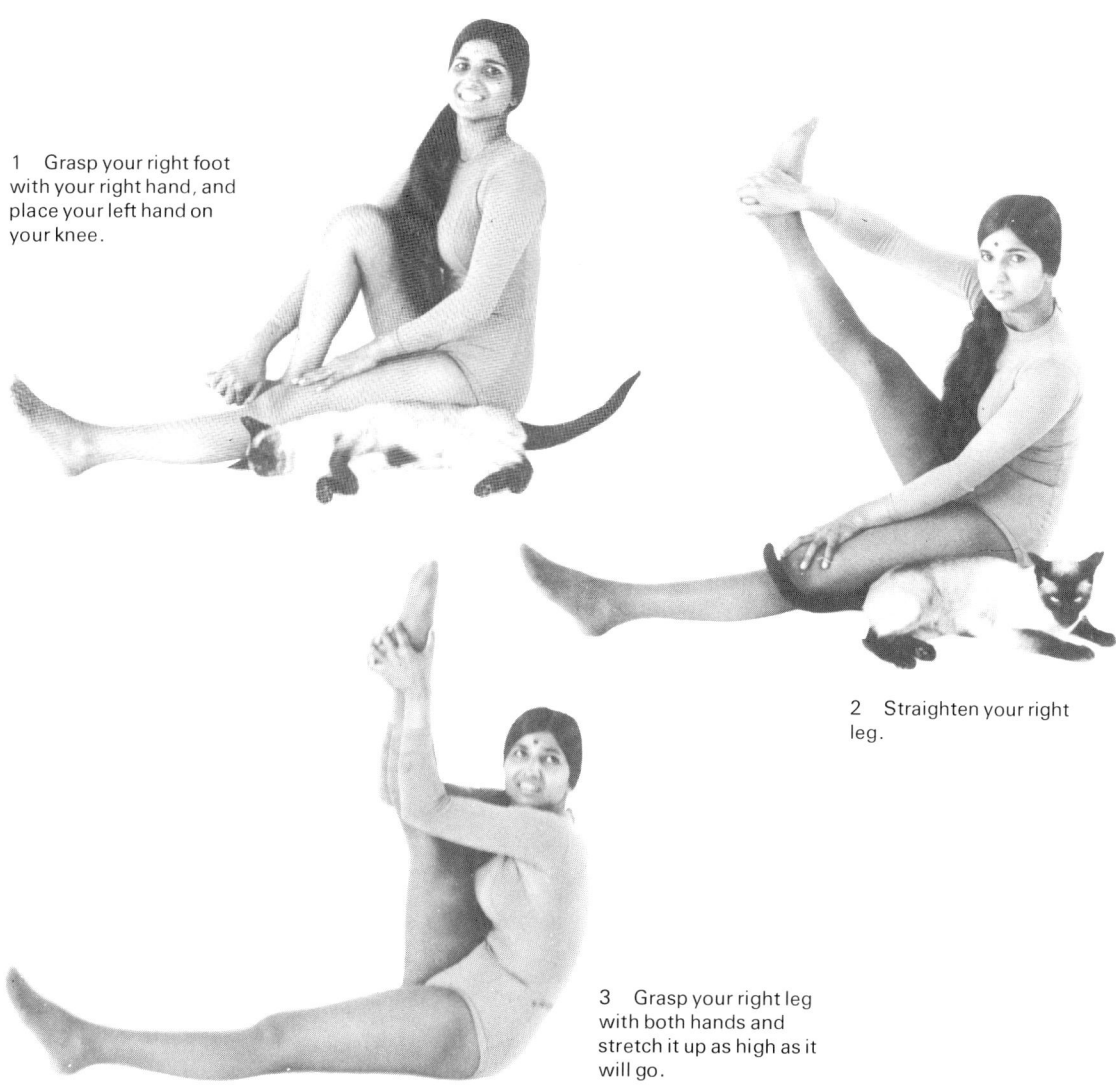

1   Grasp your right foot with your right hand, and place your left hand on your knee.

2   Straighten your right leg.

3   Grasp your right leg with both hands and stretch it up as high as it will go.

Squats

This is the best exercise you can do to develop your calves and trim your ankles.

1   Hands on your hips, feet slightly apart to give you balance, breathing in slowly, come up on your toes.

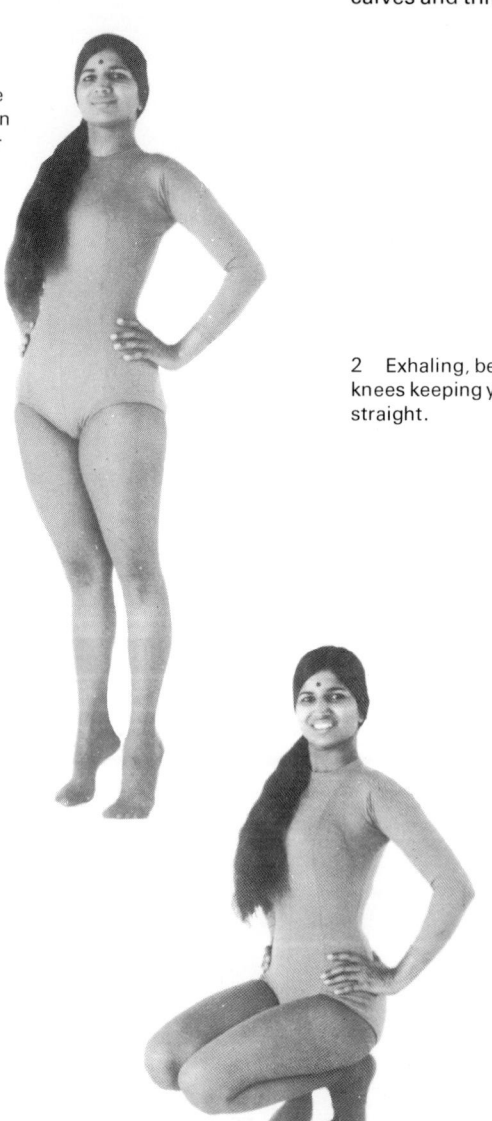

2   Exhaling, bend your knees keeping your back straight.

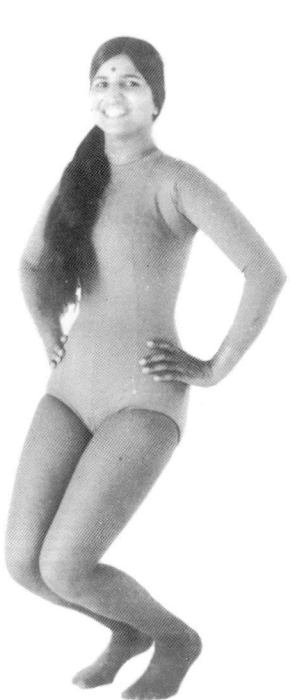

3   Without letting your heels touch the ground, try to sit on your heels.

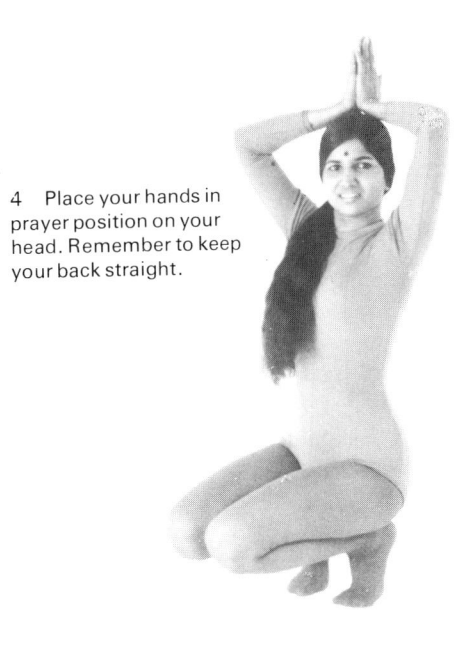

4   Place your hands in prayer position on your head. Remember to keep your back straight.

5   Breathing in, stand up slowly.

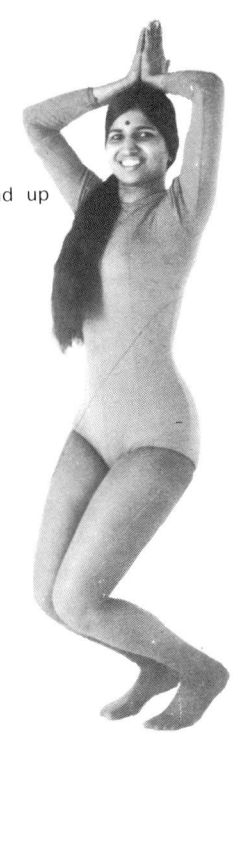

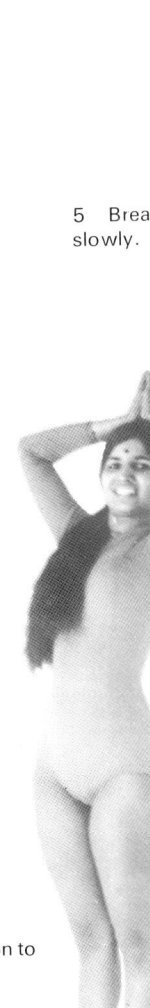

6   Stretch right up on to your toes.

7   Exhaling, drop your heels back on to the floor and relax.

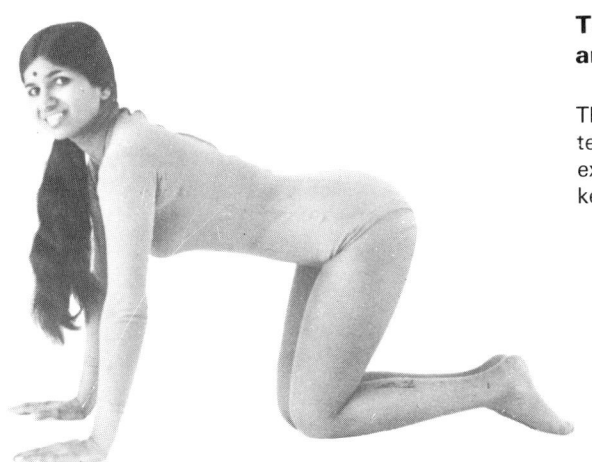

To Firm Your Buttocks, Lower Back, Hips and Thighs

The muscles of our buttocks being large and bulky tend to sag and become flabby through lack of exercise. The following postures are designed to keep your buttocks firm, taut, and well shaped.

1   Elbows straight, kneel on your hands and knees.

2   Inhaling, stretch your left leg back behind you.

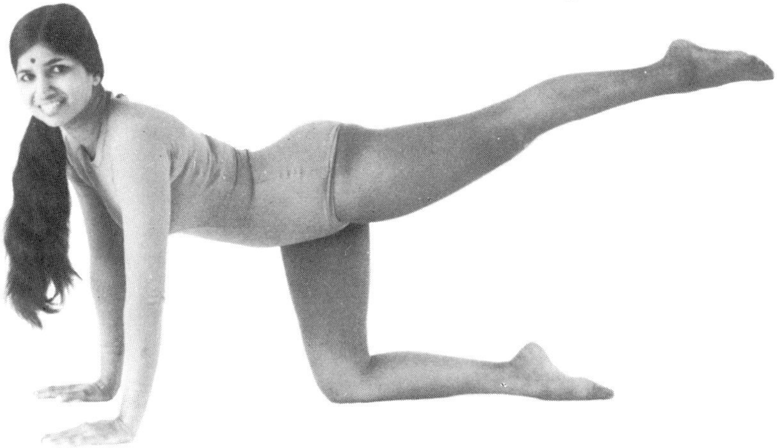

3   Exhaling, place your left knee between your hands.

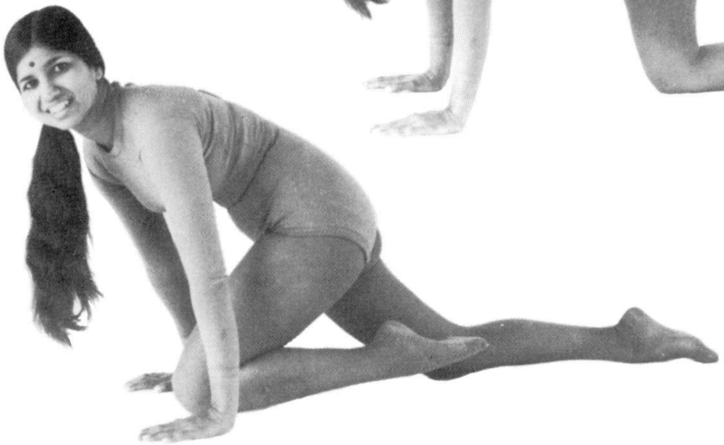

4   Inhaling, stretch your left leg back again to position 2.

5   Exhaling, place it beside your right knee (position 1), and repeat the exercise with your right leg.

Side Stretch

Apart from firming your buttocks, this exercise also massages your lower back and firms your thighs.

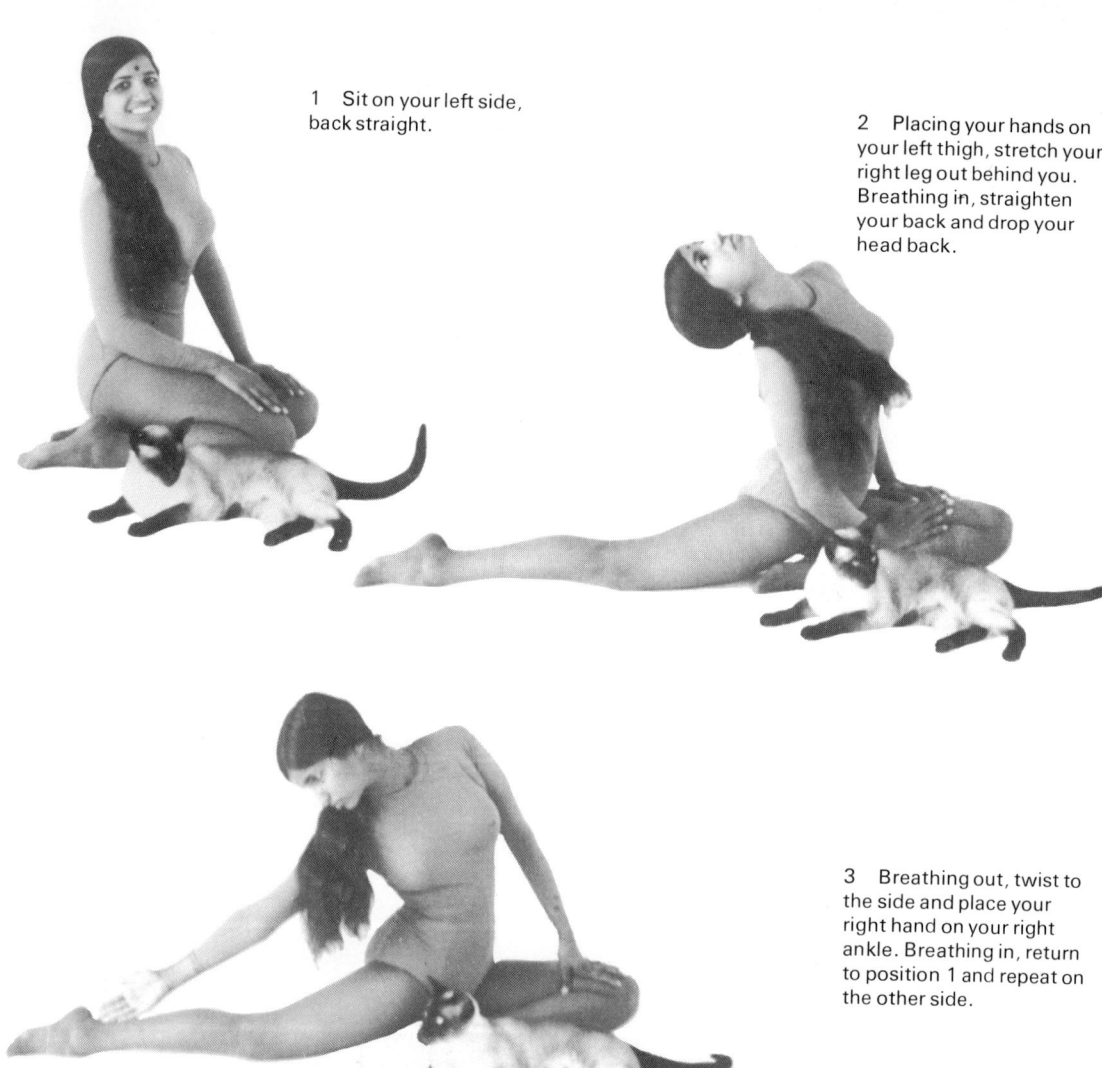

1   Sit on your left side, back straight.

2   Placing your hands on your left thigh, stretch your right leg out behind you. Breathing in, straighten your back and drop your head back.

3   Breathing out, twist to the side and place your right hand on your right ankle. Breathing in, return to position 1 and repeat on the other side.

Chakrasana (Wheel)

For the beginner

A healthy, supple and flexible spine, gives you a healthy nervous system. Chakrasana gently massages your back, calms your nerves, and helps you overcome depression.

1   Lie on your back, with your knees bent. Hands on your waist, with your thumbs in the front and fingers at the back.

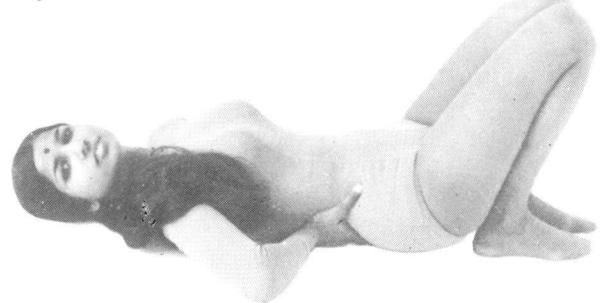

3   Breathing out, slowly return to position 1 and relax.

2   Breathing in, slowly push your buttocks up as high as you can.

This Increases the Blood Supply to the Pubic Area and Reproductive System.

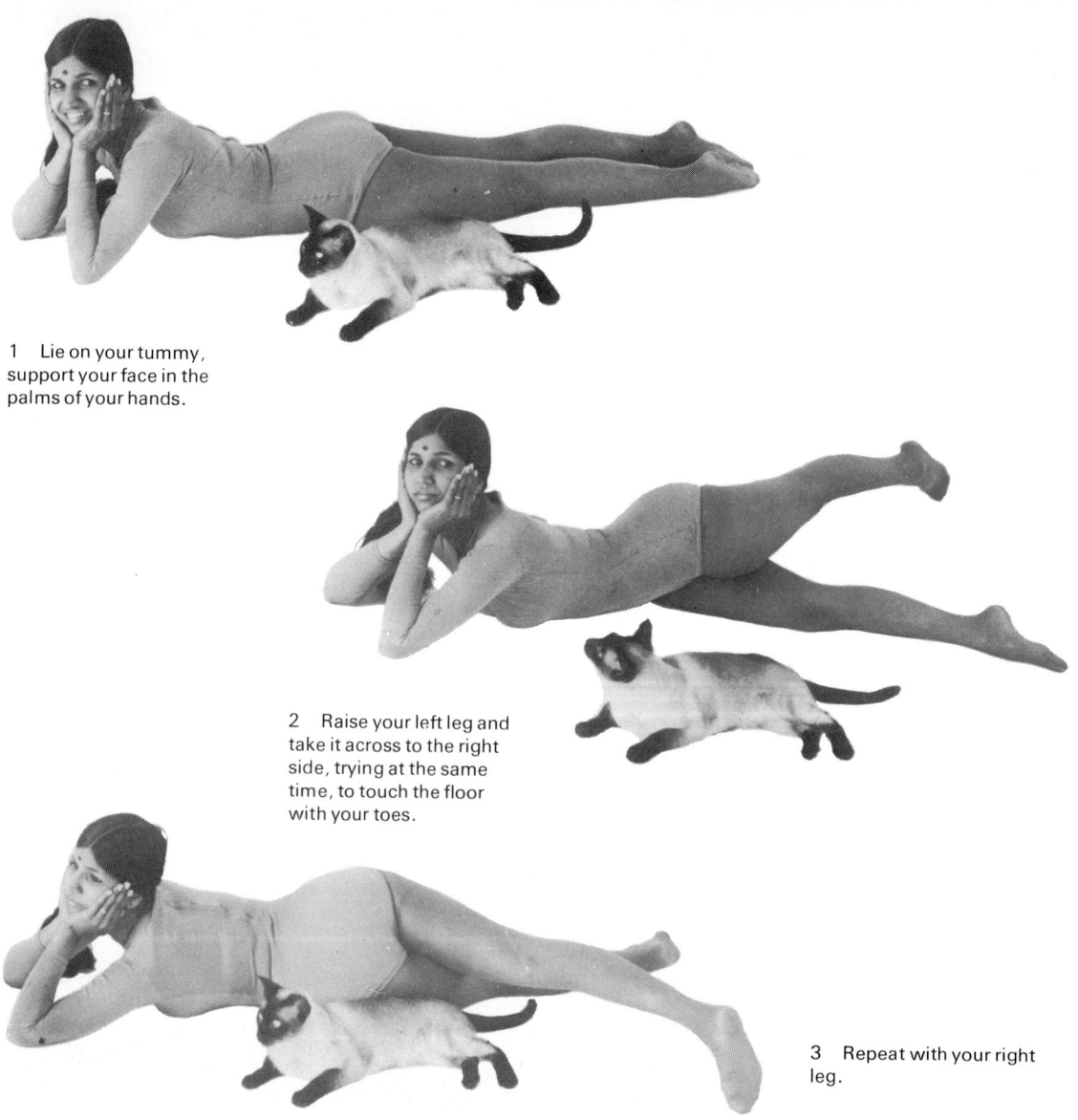

1 Lie on your tummy, support your face in the palms of your hands.

2 Raise your left leg and take it across to the right side, trying at the same time, to touch the floor with your toes.

3 Repeat with your right leg.

Ardha Dhanurasana (Half Bow)

This reduces fat around your tummy and hips. All the vertebrae of the spinal column benefit from the intense stretch. The abdominal organs receive extra blood, and tension and stiffness in your shoulders are relieved.

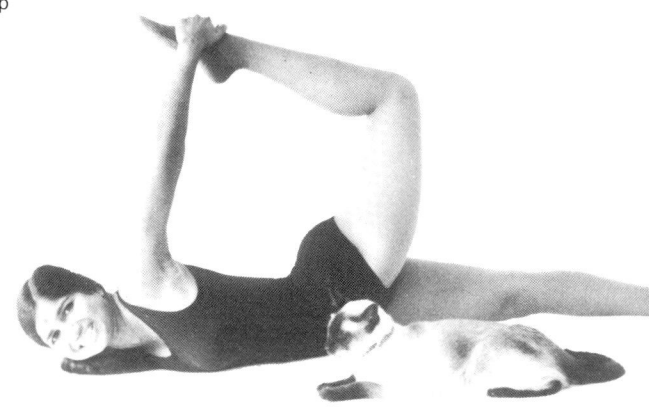

1   Lie on your tummy, bend your knee and grasp your left foot with your left hand.

2   Breathing in, slowly raise your leg as high as you can, then breathing out, gradually return to position 1, and repeat with the other leg.

3   Now, with your left hand grasp your right foot, and breathing in, raise your right leg as high as possible. Breathing in, return.

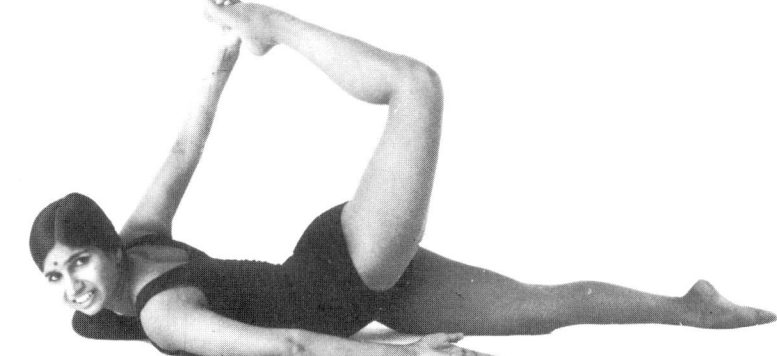

4   Repeat, using your left leg and right hand.

Salabhasana (Locust)

This strengthens and massages abdominal and back muscles. It is the major exercise to tone the lower back, kidneys and adrenal glands.

1   Lie on your tummy, hands beneath your thighs.

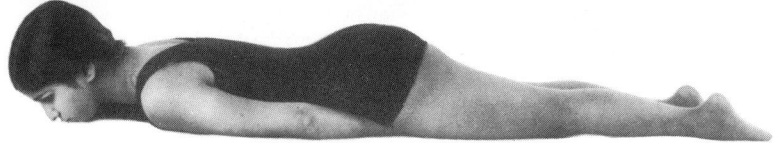

2   Breathing in, and with knees straight, raise both legs . . .

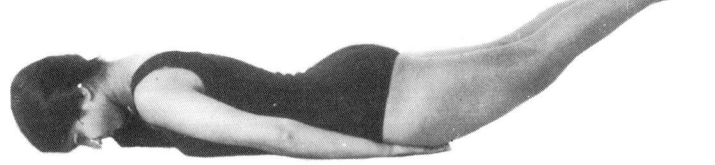

3   . . . as high as you can.

4   Breathing out, slowly lower your legs and relax.

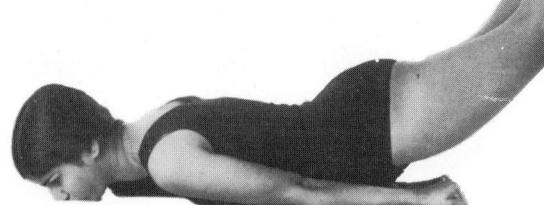

Paschimottanasana
Entire back stretch

This tones liver, spleen and the kidneys, relieving discomfort and pain during menstrual periods. You will feel the stretch from your heels to your head.

1   Sit with your back straight and arms outstretched before you. Inhale.

2   Grasp your ankles or legs.

3   If you can, grasp your feet.

4   Exhaling, take your head towards your knees and try to place your elbows on the ground.

Ardha—Matsyendrasana (Spinal Twist)

This exercise massages every vertebra in your spinal column, relieving the stiffness and tension in your back and neck. It is a must for sufferers of backache and will give you courage and inner strength.

1   Sit with knees bent, arms outstretched at either side.

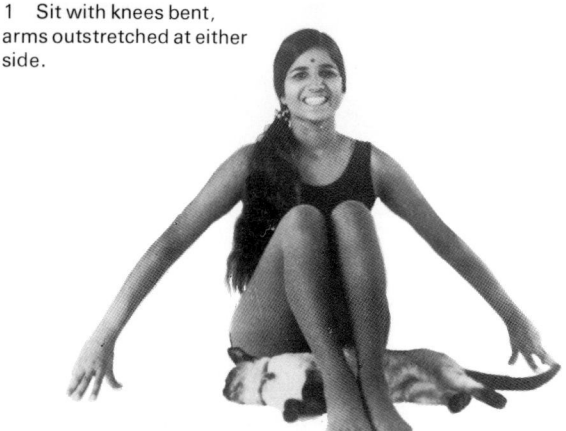

2   Place your right leg under your left thigh.

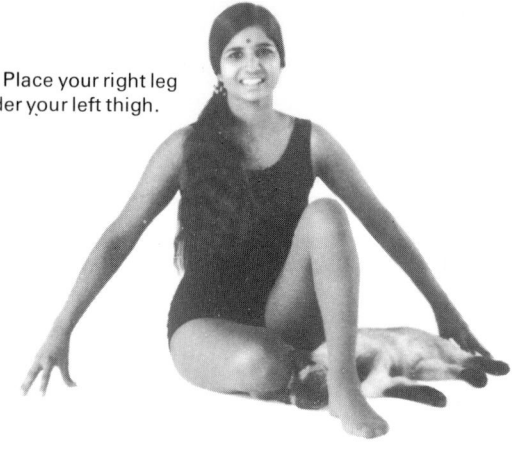

3   Now step over your left knee with your right foot.

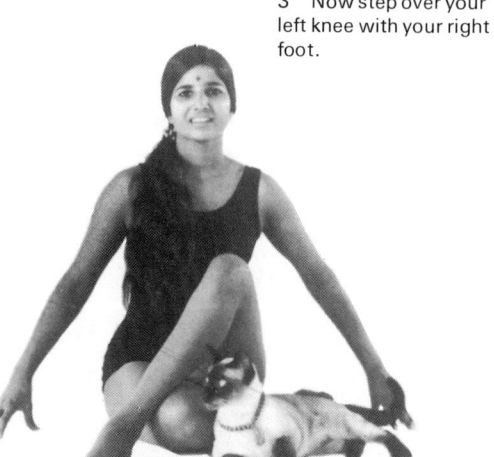

4   Grasp your left ankle with your left hand and taking your right hand behind your back, inhale and twist to the right side, so that you are looking back over your right shoulder.

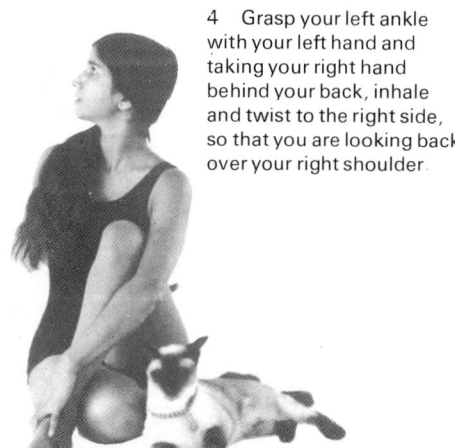

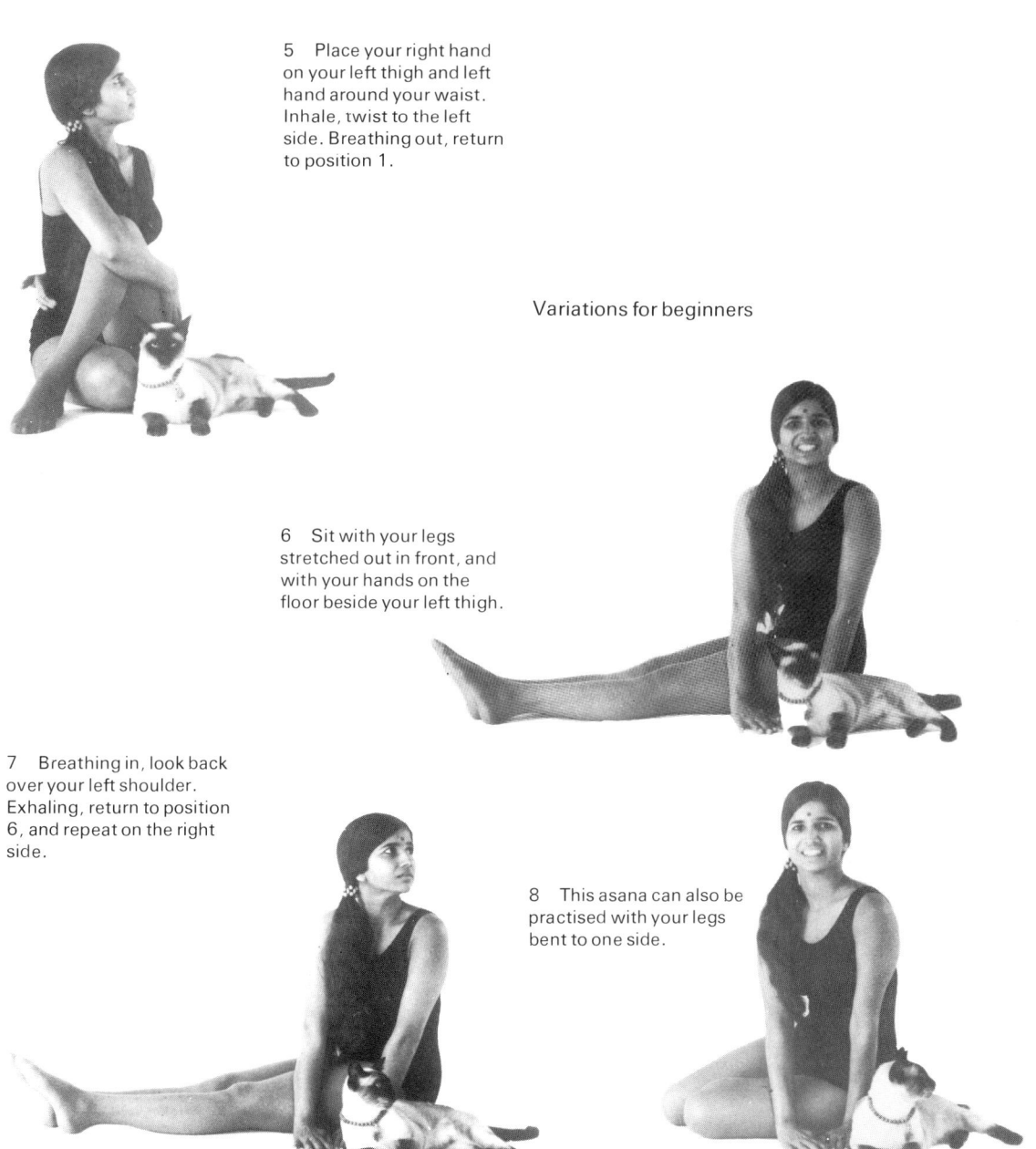

5 Place your right hand on your left thigh and left hand around your waist. Inhale, twist to the left side. Breathing out, return to position 1.

Variations for beginners

6 Sit with your legs stretched out in front, and with your hands on the floor beside your left thigh.

7 Breathing in, look back over your left shoulder. Exhaling, return to position 6, and repeat on the right side.

8 This asana can also be practised with your legs bent to one side.

The Glands

Ustrasana (Camel)

You can feel the gentle stretch in the front of your thighs, and tummy, and at the same time this massages your spine. It also massages your adrenal glands, which produce adrenalin to give you energy, and the hormones which control carbohydrate metabolism.

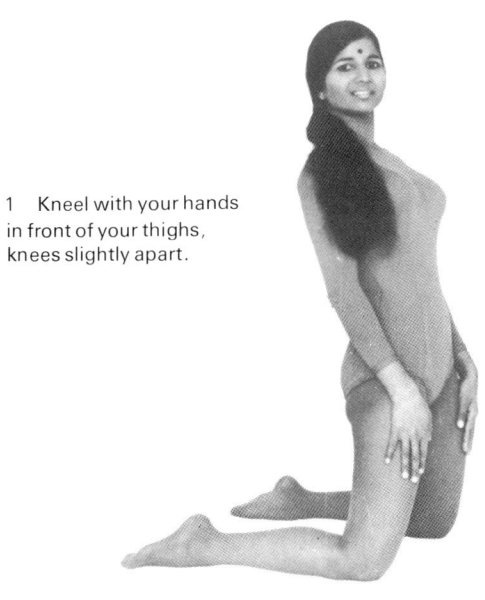

1   Kneel with your hands in front of your thighs, knees slightly apart.

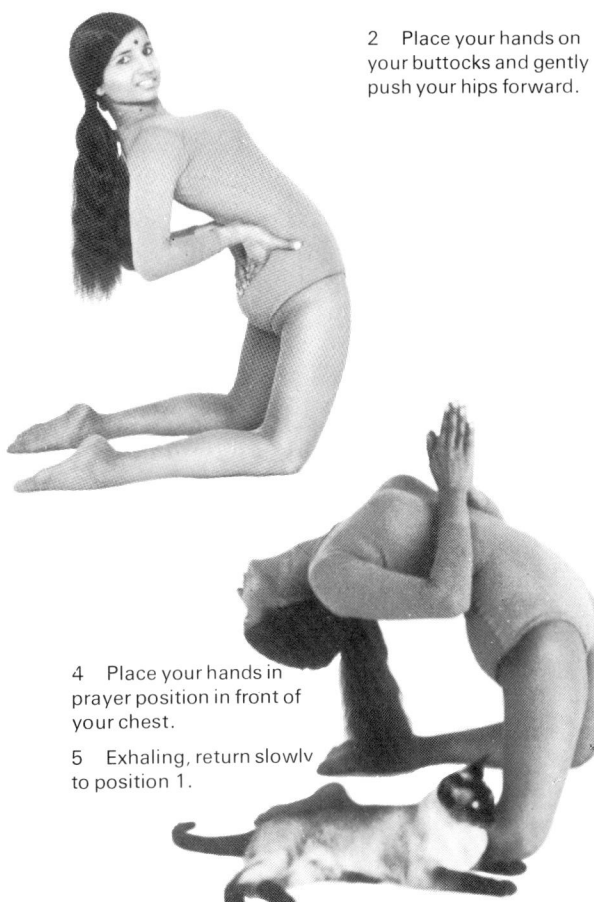

2   Place your hands on your buttocks and gently push your hips forward.

3   Inhaling, drop your head back and balance.

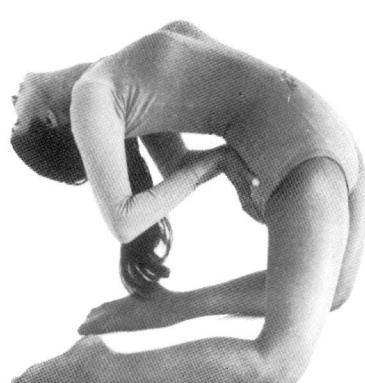

4   Place your hands in prayer position in front of your chest.

5   Exhaling, return slowly to position 1.

Sarvangasana (Shoulderstand)

The shoulderstand stimulates the thyroid and parathyroid glands. It also relieves conditions such as varicose veins and haemorrhoids, massages the nervous system and sends extra blood to your eyes, head and brain. The result is a healthy, glowing complexion, and a new vitality.

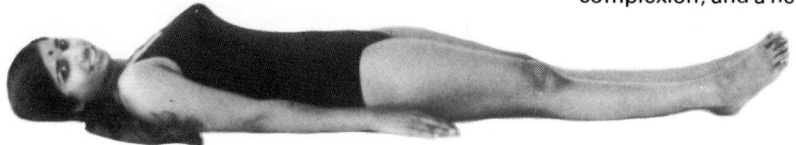

1   Lie on your back, palms firmly on the ground and toes together.

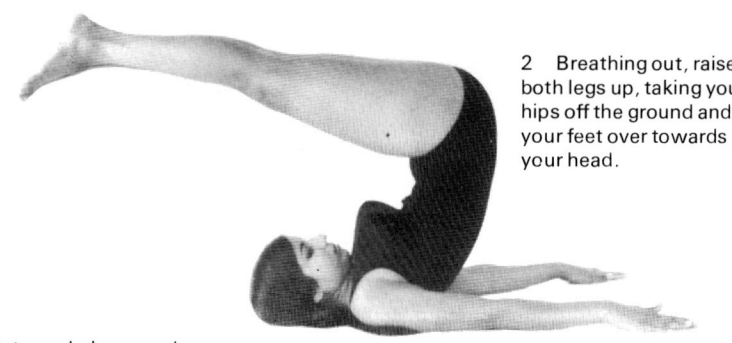

2   Breathing out, raise both legs up, taking your hips off the ground and your feet over towards your head.

3   Get your balance and support your back with your hands.

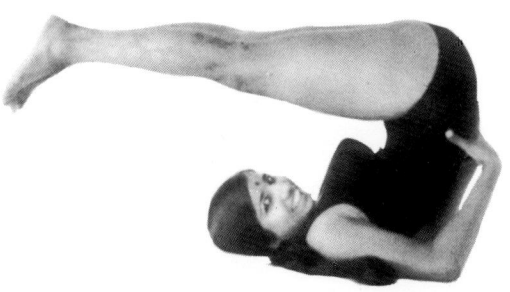

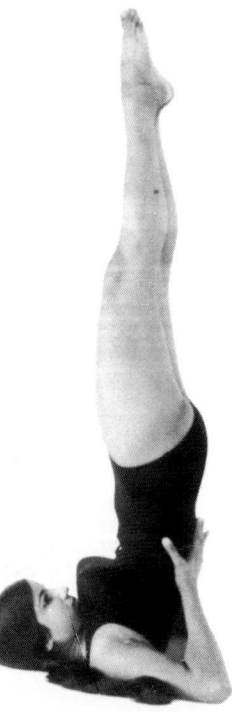

4   Slowly straighten your legs and hold this position for a count of four. Inhaling, gently return, step by step to position 2, by taking your legs towards your head, placing your hands on the ground, and then lowering firstly your body and then your legs to the ground.

Janusirasana
Head to knee posture

This exercise aids digestion and massages all the tummy organs including the pancreas, which produces insulin to regulate the metabolism of sugar.

1   Sit with your right leg bent (right foot against your left thigh), left leg stretched out straight, and hands on your knees. Take three slow, deep breaths.

2   Bend to the left side and grasp your left ankle, toes or foot.

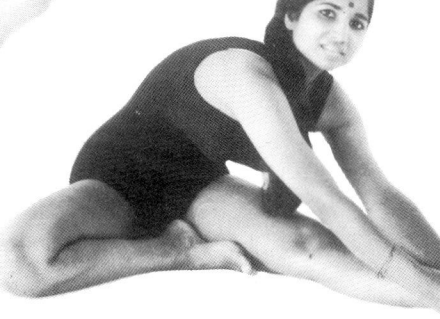

3   Exhale and take your head down to your knee.

4   Inhaling, return to position 1 and repeat with the other leg.

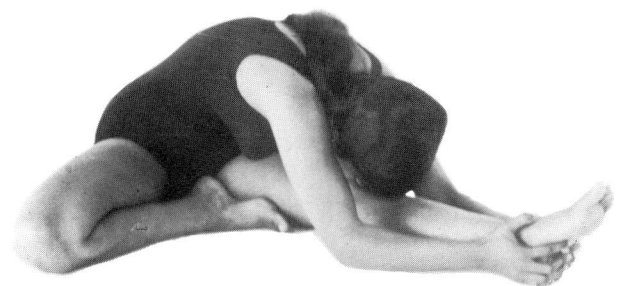

Dhanurasana (The Bow)

An asana which stimulates your entire body through its action on the adrenal glands. It invigorates spinal nerves and gives elasticity to your spine, while increasing the supply of the blood to the abdomen.

1   Lie on your tummy, bend your knees and grasp your ankles.

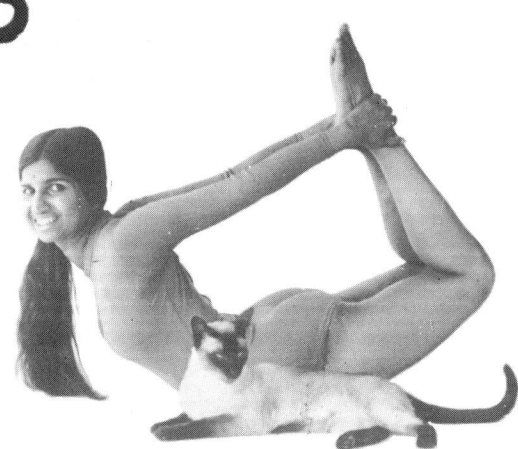

2   Breathing in, slowly raise your head and shoulders off the floor. At the same time, pull your ankles up, so that your body forms a bow.

3   Breathing out, slowly lower yourself to the floor and relax.

Balance

Balance, like many of the other senses, deteriorates with age. This is why so many elderly folk injure themselves through falls. By practising balancing we can restore our co-ordination, and gain poise, grace and self-confidence.

Pelvic Balance

1   Sit with your knees bent, hands clasped beneath your knees.

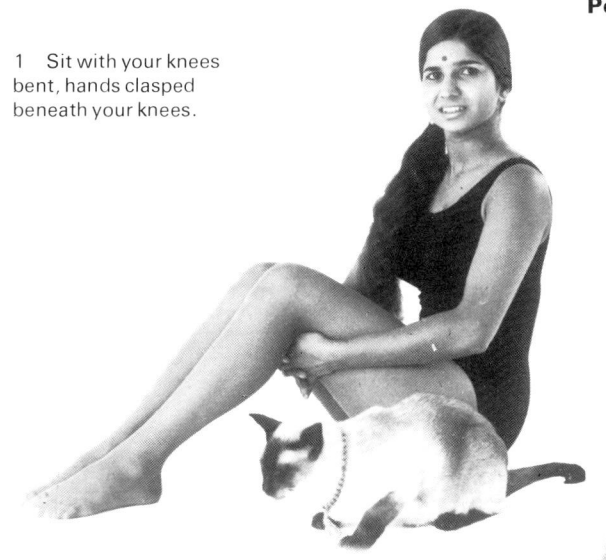

2   Slowly raise your feet off the ground and straighten your knees. Balance for a count of four, before lowering your legs to the floor.

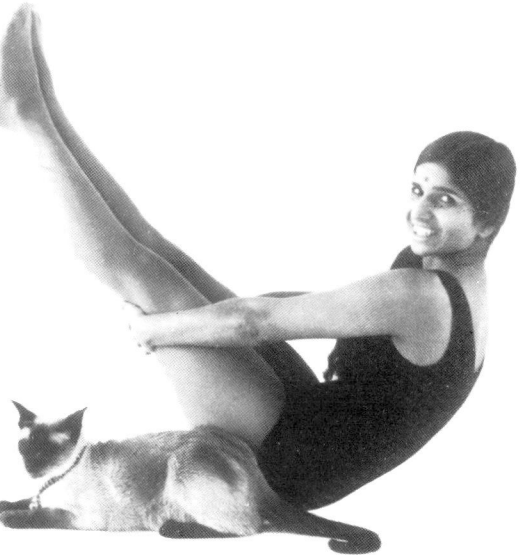

Natarajasana (Dancing posture)

This gives you confidence, poise and grace, reduces fat around your hips and upper thighs, and strengthens your legs.

1   Stand on your right leg and grasp your left foot with your left hand. Right hand stretched out in front.

2   Breathing in, slowly raise your left leg.

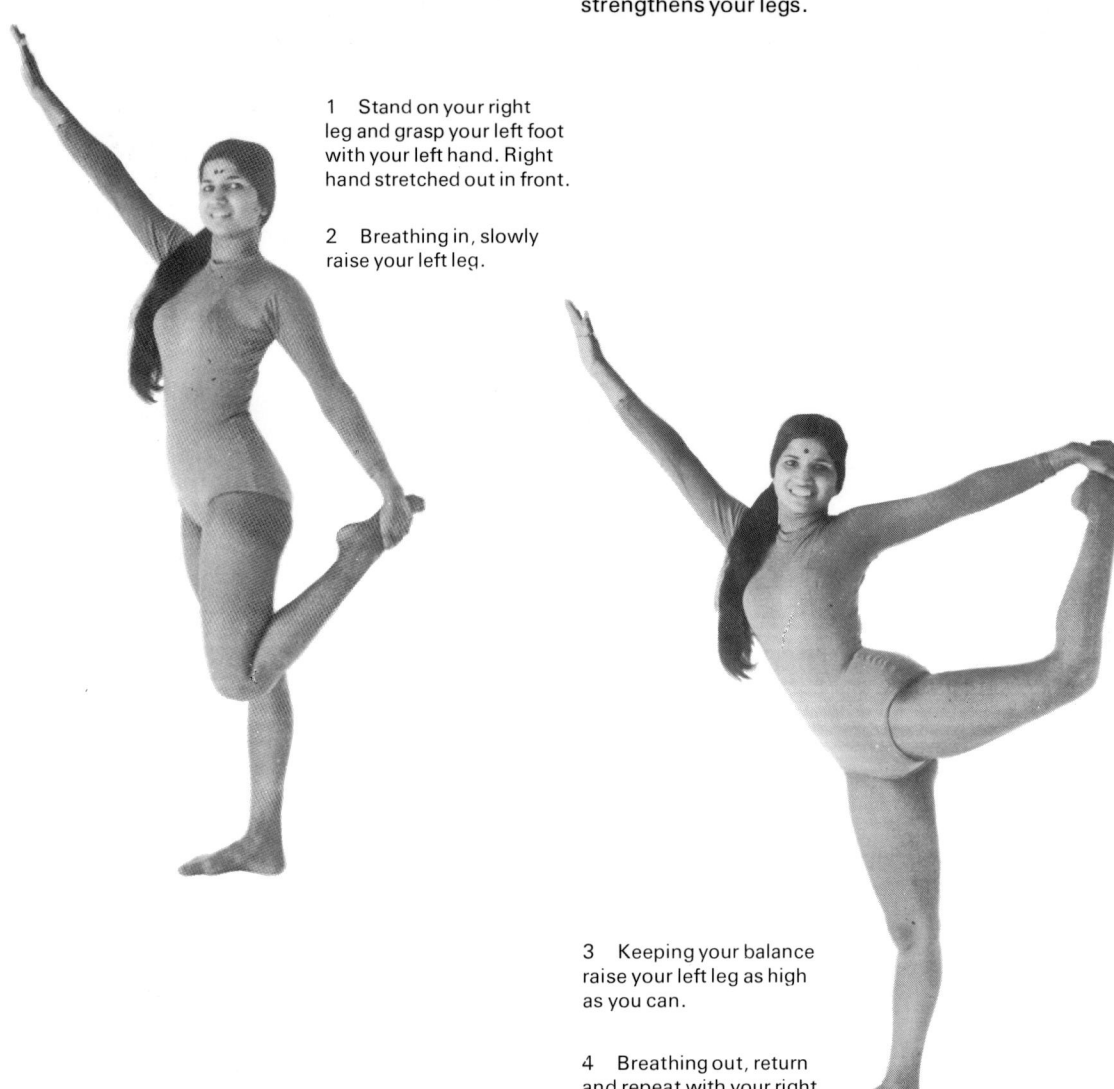

3   Keeping your balance raise your left leg as high as you can.

4   Breathing out, return and repeat with your right leg.

Stork

To improve your powers of attention and concentration.

1   Stand on your right leg and place your left foot on your right knee. Beginners, practise this first step, until you can stand perfectly steady.

2   Slowly lift your left foot up towards your groin, as high as you can.

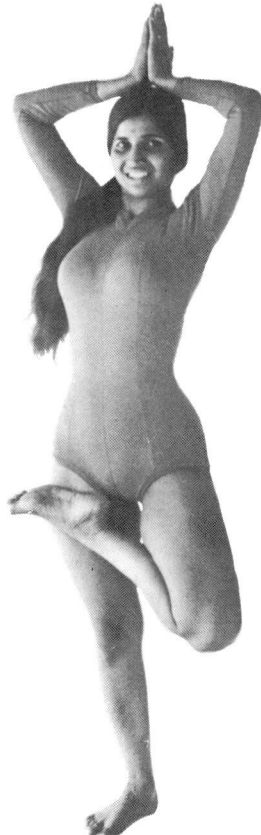

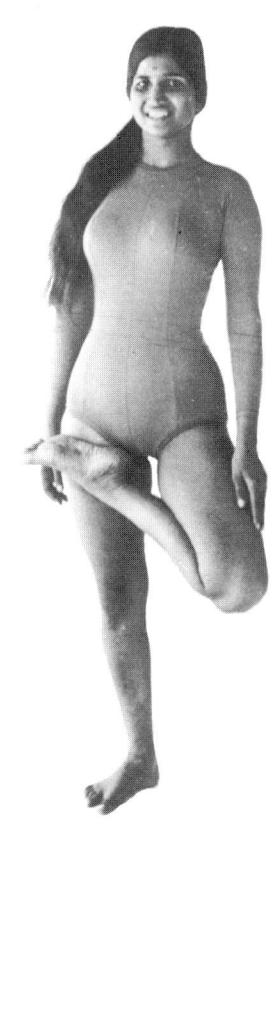

3   Breathing in, place your hands in prayer position above your head. Balance for a complete breath. Breathing out, return and repeat on your left leg.

The Flying Balance

This improves harmony of body and mind. By learning to balance firmly on the sole of one foot, you can maintain physical and mental equilibrium.

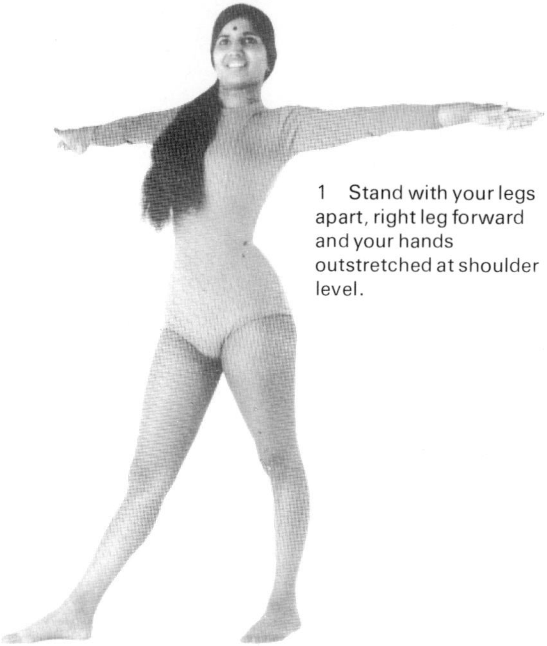

1   Stand with your legs apart, right leg forward and your hands outstretched at shoulder level.

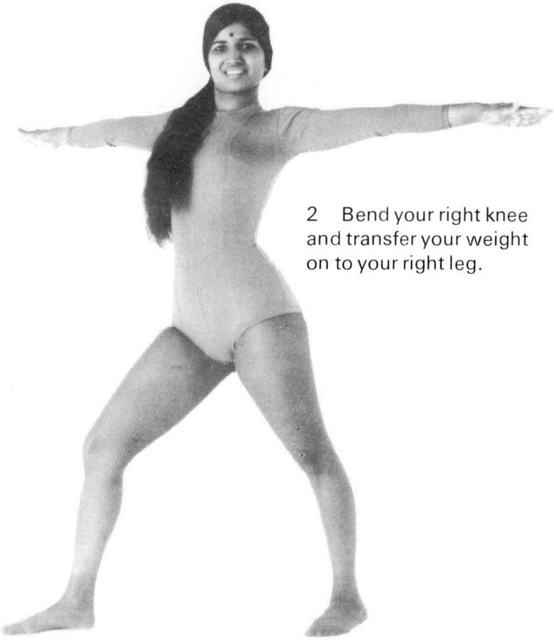

2   Bend your right knee and transfer your weight on to your right leg.

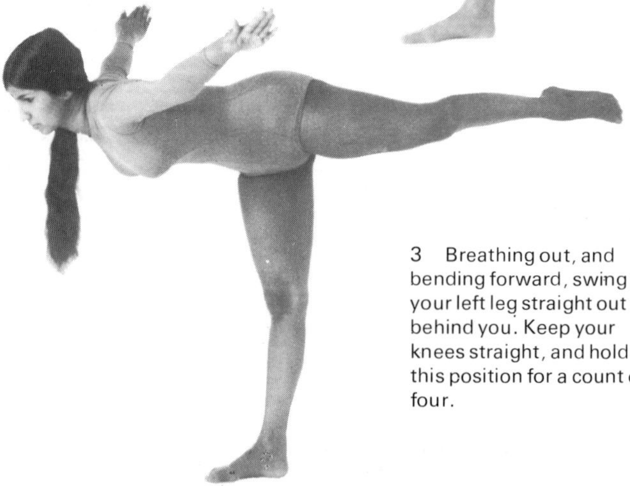

3   Breathing out, and bending forward, swing your left leg straight out behind you. Keep your knees straight, and hold this position for a count of four.

4   Inhaling, slowly return and repeat with your other leg.

Pregnancy

Breathing, relaxation and postures will tone the pelvic muscles and ensure easy labour.

Cat Hump

Before child-birth, the Cat Hump will relieve lower back pain. Practised after child-birth, it will tighten your tummy muscles.

2   Exhaling, drop your head forward and pull your tummy in as far as you can. Arch your back at the same time.

1   Kneel on your hands and knees.

3   Inhaling, lift your head up and push your tummy down.

Ideal for Pregnancy, this keeps Everyone's Knees in Good Shape as well.

1   Sit between your feet, hands on your hips.

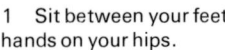

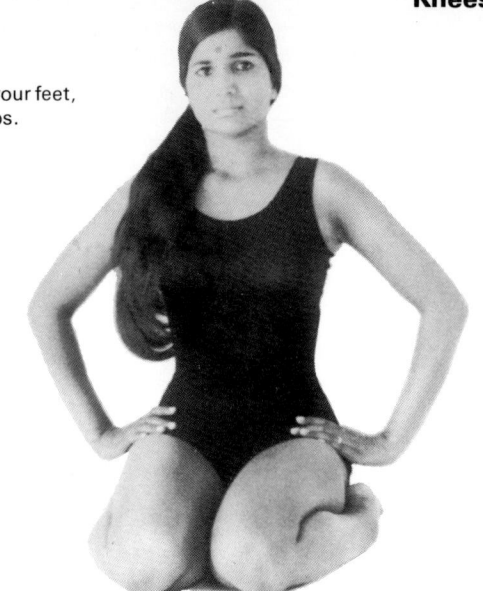

2   Breathing in, spread your knees as wide as you can . . .

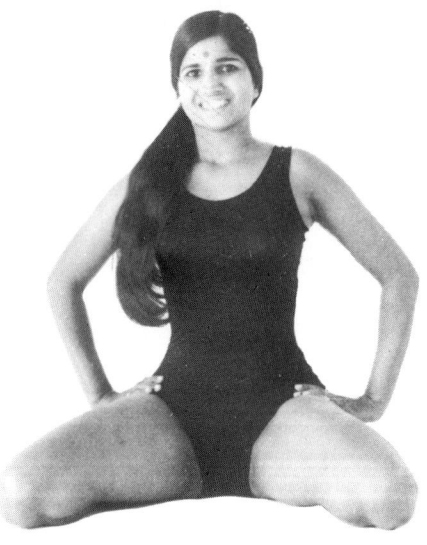

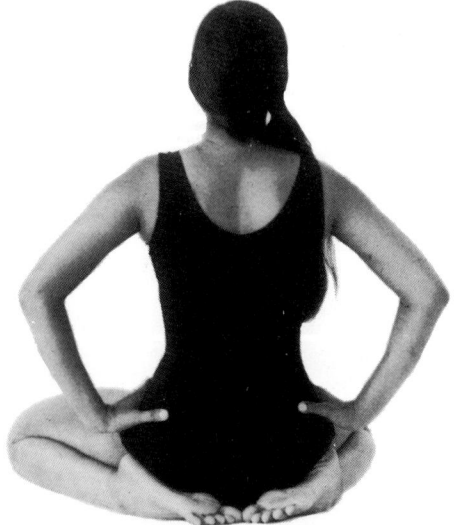

3   . . . trying to touch your toes behind your back.

4   Breathing out, slowly bring your knees together and relax.

For Pelvic Flexibility in Pregnancy

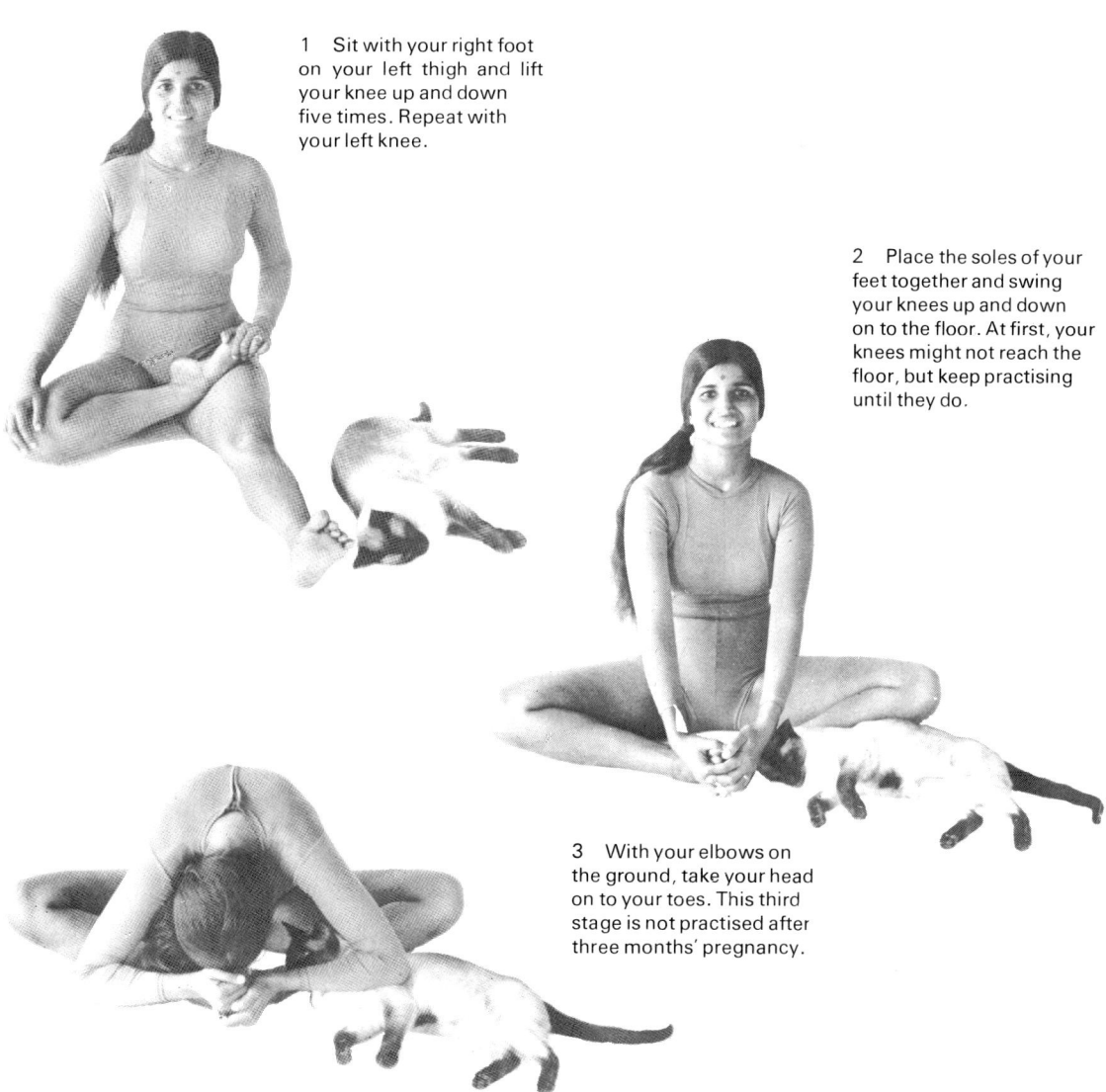

1 Sit with your right foot on your left thigh and lift your knee up and down five times. Repeat with your left knee.

2 Place the soles of your feet together and swing your knees up and down on to the floor. At first, your knees might not reach the floor, but keep practising until they do.

3 With your elbows on the ground, take your head on to your toes. This third stage is not practised after three months' pregnancy.

Constipation, Asthma,
Varicose Veins and Sore Throats

Constipation

Stomach Contractions

This is always practised on an empty stomach. Women who are pregnant or who are having their menstrual period should avoid practising it. The muscle contraction tones the abdominal muscles, improves digestion and gives freedom from constipation. It also trims your tummy.

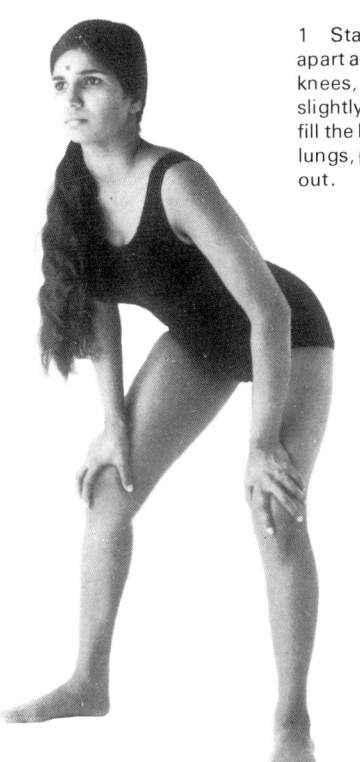

1   Stand with your feet apart and hands on your knees, which should be slightly bent. Breathing in, fill the lower part of your lungs, pushing your tummy out.

2   Breathing out, empty the lower part of your lungs, contracting your abdominal muscles up and back.

Note:
Avoid overcooked and processed foods. Eat fresh fruits and salads for extra roughage. Apples with skin, spinach and onions also help to relieve constipation.

Asthma

Matsyasana (Fish)

This tones up the nerves which have their roots in the solar plexus region. It greatly assists breathing too.

1 Sit cross-legged or in lotus position, hands on your knees.

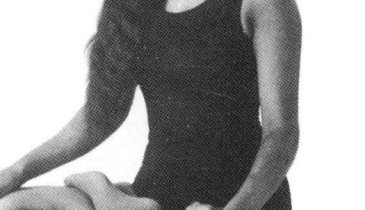

2 Breathing in, lean back slowly until the top of your head is resting on the floor. Your back should be arched.

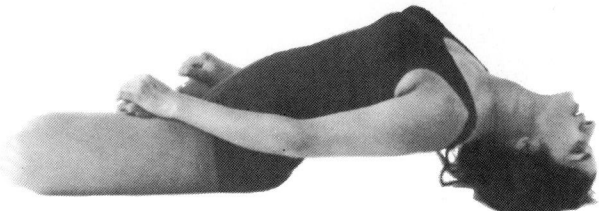

3 Place your hands in prayer position in front of your chest. Hold for a while and breathing out, gently return to position 1 and relax.

4 Beginners can do this exercise with their legs stretched out straight.

Complete Chest Expansion

Practised with eyes closed, this exercise induces calmness and tranquility. This is most important for asthmatics whose attacks are often triggered by emotional upset.

All adult asthma sufferers should practise relaxation and meditation.

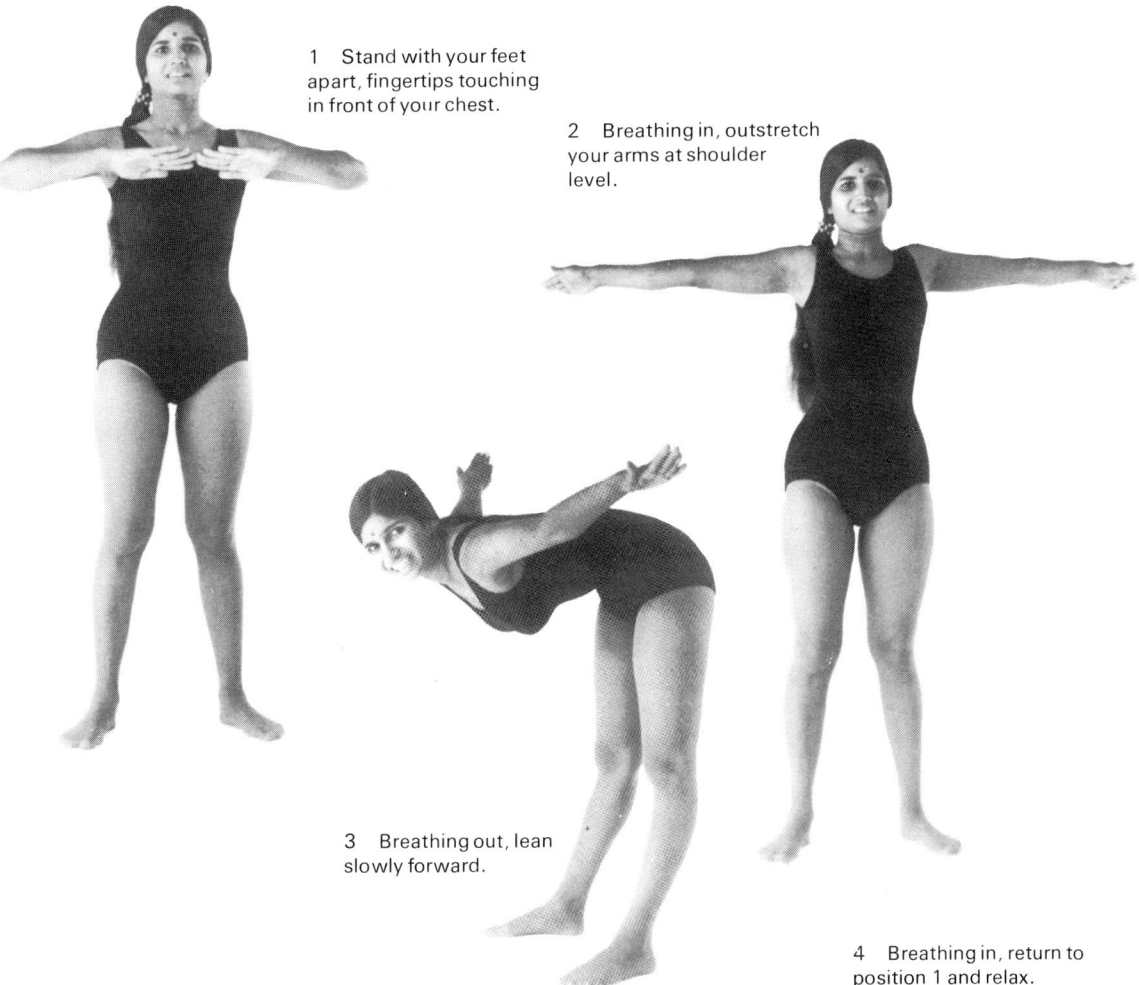

1   Stand with your feet apart, fingertips touching in front of your chest.

2   Breathing in, outstretch your arms at shoulder level.

3   Breathing out, lean slowly forward.

4   Breathing in, return to position 1 and relax.

Varicose Veins

Varicose vein sufferers should practise all the inverted postures given in this book, and avail themselves of every opportunity to put their legs up on a chair or cushion to aid the return of blood to the body.

1   Lie on your back with your hands by your sides and raise your legs until they form a right angle with your body.

2   Point your toes down towards your chest.

3   Slowly bend your left leg, by taking your knee down to your chest, and then straighten it. Now bend and straighten your right leg. Repeat at least five times with each leg.

Sore Throat

Simhasana (Lion Posture)

A very good exercise to smooth the tension lines from your face. Cures sore throat and bad breath and stimulates the larynx. After practising this pose for a while, you will find your voice becomes clearer.

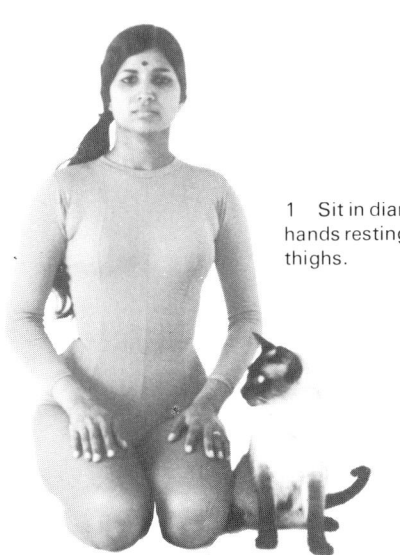

1 Sit in diamond posture, hands resting on your thighs.

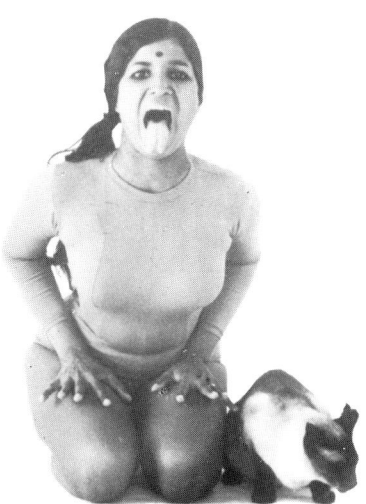

2 Breathing out, press your hands on your thighs, spread your fingers wide, push your tongue out and open your eyes as wide as you can.

3 Breathing in, relax.

Relaxation

Relaxation

We must apply yoga relaxation to our daily lives to overcome insomnia, chronic fatigue, headaches, eye strain, neck pain and backaches. These and a thousand more troubles can be caused through tension.

1 Sit in diamond posture, hands loosely by your sides.

2 Exhaling, lean forward and place your head on the ground.

3 Lift your buttocks off your heels. Breathe in and out as you please, but slowly.

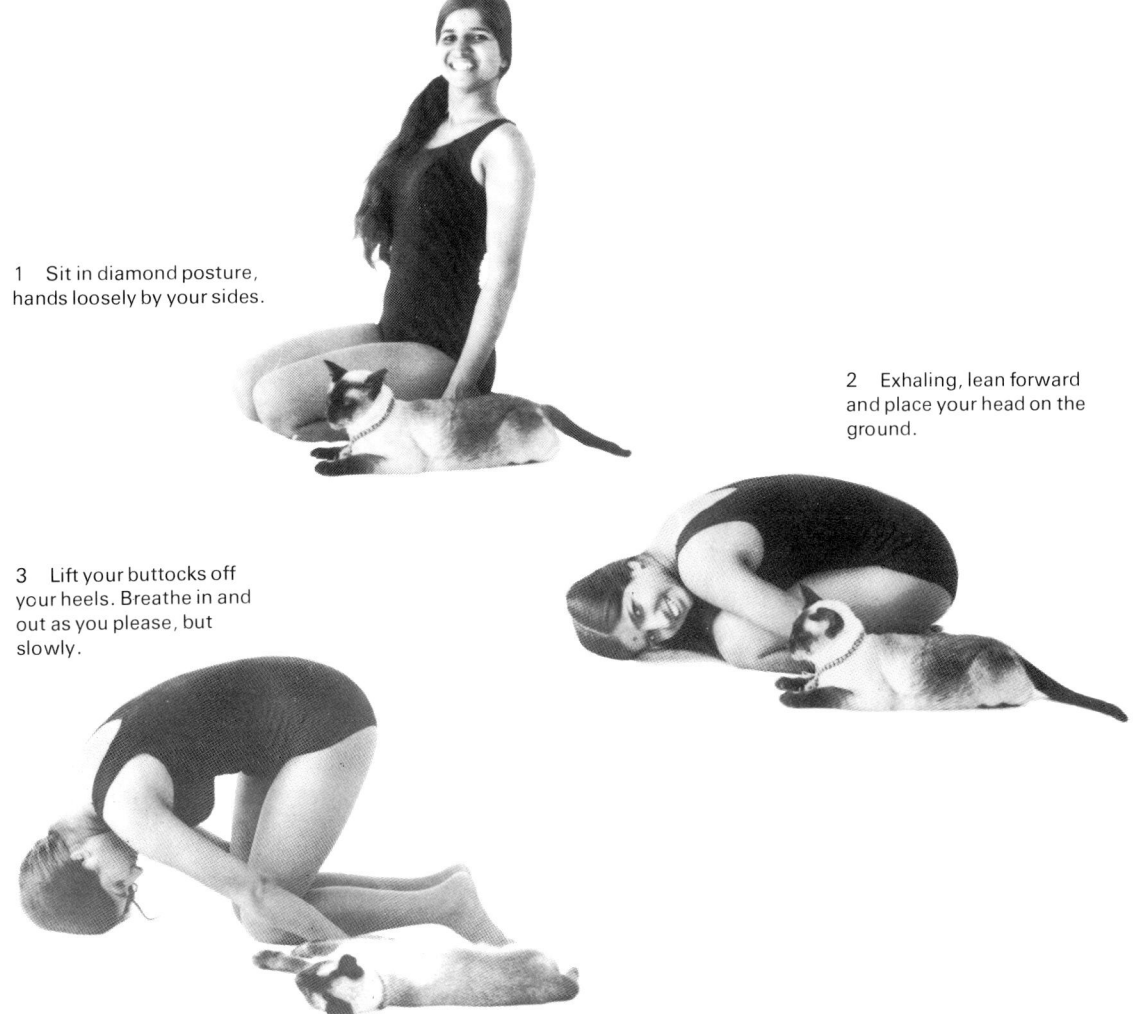

4   Straighten your knees.

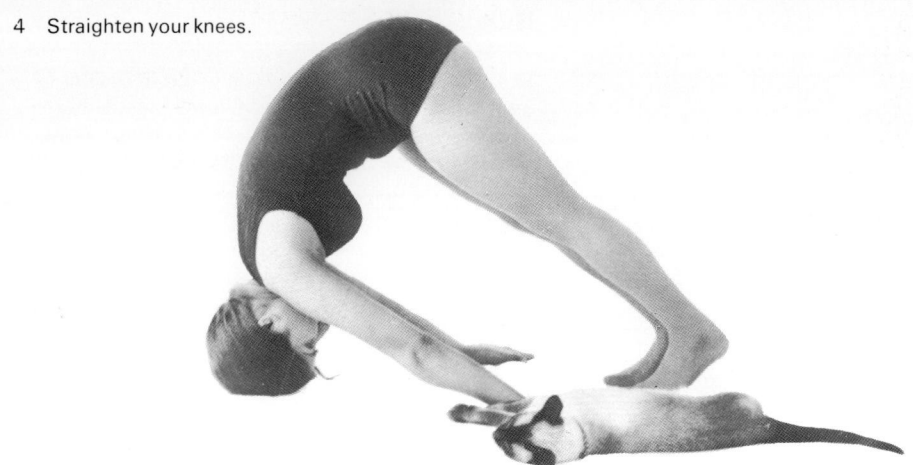

Variation

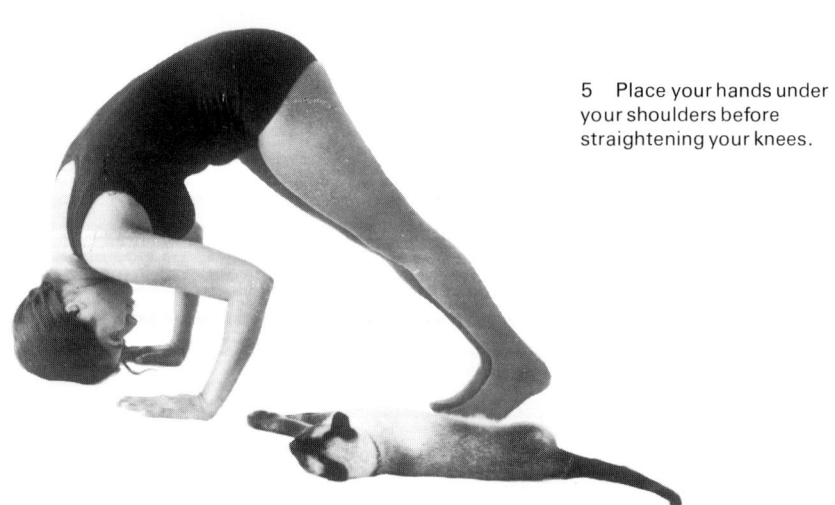

5   Place your hands under
your shoulders before
straightening your knees.

6   Exhaling, slowly return
to position 1, close your
eyes and relax for a few
seconds.

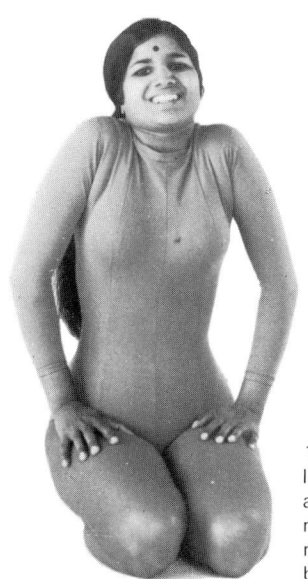

Shoulder Shrugging

This simple exercise relieves tension headaches, and strain at the base of your neck.

1   Sit in diamond posture, lift your shoulders as high as possible, and gently massage your neck by moving your shoulders backward and forward.

Sanmuki Mudra

To overcome negative thoughts and conflicting emotions.

1   Place your thumbs in your ears, index fingers on your eyelids, second fingers on your nostrils, third fingers on your upper lip, and your small fingers on your lower lip.

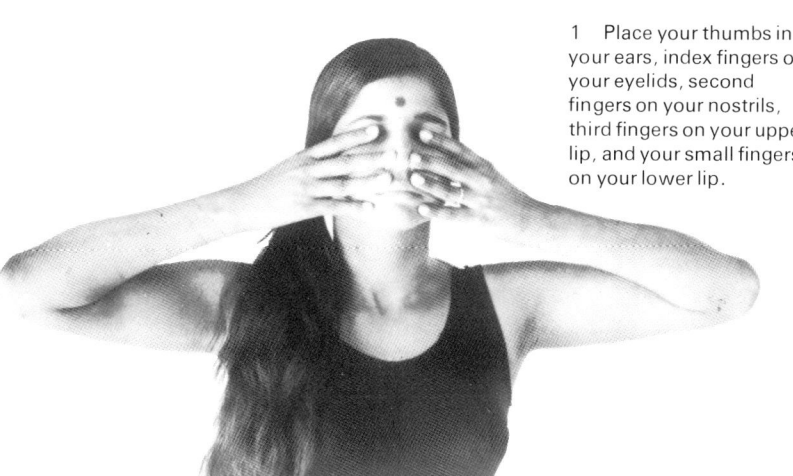

2   Open your nostrils, inhale, hold your breath for a count of four and breathe out.

Savasana (Complete Relaxation Posture)

1 Lie on your back, heels together, feet apart, hands by your sides and your chin lowered slightly towards your body. Your mouth should be closed, with your tongue touching your upper teeth.

2 Half close your eyes and concentrate on the area between your eye brows or on your deep, slow, rhythmic breathing.

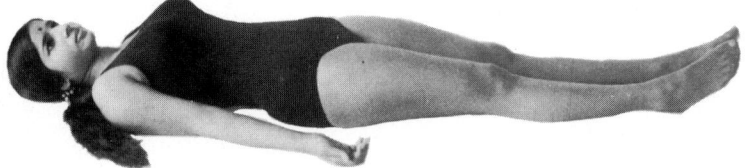

After reading this book we should resolve to tackle all our daily problems with a calm and positive outlook, to rise above pettiness, jealousy and anxiety and to refuse to let them disturb our inner peace.

Weight Reducing Hints

1   If you are just a little overweight, a few weeks of avoiding sweets, cakes, soft drinks and second helpings will soon trim you down. But if you are many pounds overweight, then prepare yourself for a three month effort. Set yourself a reasonable goal; eat your normal fare—just eat less. You will lose at least one pound a week consistently.

2   Many dieters become frustrated if their scales don't show a dramatic loss within the first few days and such people could follow a fast. All religions have taught fasting which helps the body as well as the mind. Begin with a short fast—a glass of fresh vegetable or fruit juice to replace lunch or supper. Try going to bed without supper and then, as the body adjusts, start a one day fast, restricting yourself to fluids only (milk, juices or weak tea). When fasting be positive. Ask God's help to cleanse and purify your body and mind, and to give you the strength to eat more moderately and sensibly. Remember, fasting is useless if you over eat the next day.

3   Avoid all sugar and flour, and everything containing either of these ingredients. Satisfy your appetite with clear soup in winter, and fresh salads in summer. Substitute fresh fruits for sweets and cakes.

4   Keep a DIET DIARY: Write down everything you eat and drink during the day and list the quantities. Everything . . . no matter how small an amount it might be. At the end of the day, you will have a record which will amaze and shame you. Insist that your husband or wife check it every night.

5   Train yourself to eat less food. Take smaller servings and no second helpings. You will be hungry at first . . . but your stomach will soon adjust and you'll find you want less.

6   Keep out of the kitchen (especially when you are bored or depressed).

7   Don't look in cake shop windows—study the new, slim fashions in the dress shops instead.

8   Reward yourself in ways that don't include food . . . a new perfume, cosmetic or piece of jewellery.

9   Keep busy all day. Spring clean, take up charity work, telephone a friend and have a long talk, and participate in a sport with your family.

10   If you are an emotional eater, then practise deep breathing and yoga. Stretch your body as often as possible, and stretch out your knotted nerves and muscles. Meditate daily with the help of your Meditation Beads and develop your willpower. Overweight is unnecessary and endangers your health and the welfare of your family.